HUMAN ANATOMY AND PHYSIOLOGY

SCOLIOSIS

CAUSES, SYMPTOMS AND TREATMENT

Human Anatomy and Physiology

Additional books in this series can be found on Nova's website under the Series tab.

Additional e-books in this series can be found on Nova's website under the e-book tab.

Physiology - Laboratory and Clinical Research

Additional books in this series can be found on Nova's website under the Series tab.

Additional e-books in this series can be found on Nova's website under the e-book tab.

HUMAN ANATOMY AND PHYSIOLOGY

SCOLIOSIS

CAUSES, SYMPTOMS AND TREATMENT

ABSOLON BESSETTE
AND
CORALIE M. ROUSSEAU
EDITORS

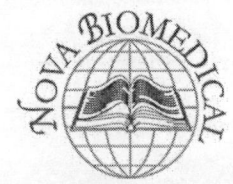

Nova Science Publishers, Inc.
New York

Copyright © 2012 by Nova Science Publishers, Inc.

All rights reserved. No part of this book may be reproduced, stored in a retrieval system or transmitted in any form or by any means: electronic, electrostatic, magnetic, tape, mechanical photocopying, recording or otherwise without the written permission of the Publisher.

For permission to use material from this book please contact us:
Telephone 631-231-7269; Fax 631-231-8175
Web Site: http://www.novapublishers.com

NOTICE TO THE READER

The Publisher has taken reasonable care in the preparation of this book, but makes no expressed or implied warranty of any kind and assumes no responsibility for any errors or omissions. No liability is assumed for incidental or consequential damages in connection with or arising out of information contained in this book. The Publisher shall not be liable for any special, consequential, or exemplary damages resulting, in whole or in part, from the readers' use of, or reliance upon, this material. Any parts of this book based on government reports are so indicated and copyright is claimed for those parts to the extent applicable to compilations of such works.

Independent verification should be sought for any data, advice or recommendations contained in this book. In addition, no responsibility is assumed by the publisher for any injury and/or damage to persons or property arising from any methods, products, instructions, ideas or otherwise contained in this publication.

This publication is designed to provide accurate and authoritative information with regard to the subject matter covered herein. It is sold with the clear understanding that the Publisher is not engaged in rendering legal or any other professional services. If legal or any other expert assistance is required, the services of a competent person should be sought. FROM A DECLARATION OF PARTICIPANTS JOINTLY ADOPTED BY A COMMITTEE OF THE AMERICAN BAR ASSOCIATION AND A COMMITTEE OF PUBLISHERS.

Additional color graphics may be available in the e-book version of this book.

Library of Congress Cataloging-in-Publication Data

Library of Congress Control Number: 2012931078

ISBN: 978-1-62081-007-1

Published by Nova Science Publishers, Inc. † New York

Contents

Preface		vii
Chapter I	Scoliosis: Causes, Genetics, Symptoms, and Treatment in a Southern Italy Population *T. Esposito, B. Varriale, G. F. DiMartino, M. Chierchia, A. Gironi Carnevale and D. Ronca*	1
Chapter II	Scoliosis, Orthodontics and Occlusion, Are There Evidence? *Amat Philippe*	49
Chapter III	Shadow Moiré Technique to Measure Deformity of the Trunk Surface in the Elderly: A Population-based Study *Flávia Porto, Jonas Lírio Gurgel, Thais Russomano and Paulo de Tarso Veras Farinatti*	73
Chapter IV	Scoliosis: Causes, Symptoms and Treatment *Reuben C.C. Soh and Hwan Tak Hee*	91
Chapter V	A New Physical Therapy Intervention for Scoliosis *Clare Lewis*	105
Chapter VI	Effects of Load Carriage on Children with Scoliosis *Daniel Hung-kay Chow and Alon Lai*	119

Chapter VII	The Pineal Gland, Melatonin and Scoliosis *Gregory Day and Bruce McPhee*	**137**
Index		**161**

Preface

Scoliosis is a lateral spinal deformity often coupled with vertebral rotation with most of the cases presenting as idiopathic. In this book, the authors present topical research in the study of the causes, symptoms and treatment of scoliosis. Topics discussed include the history and classification of scoliosis; the connection between idiopathic scoliosis, orthodontics and occlusion and their therapeutic implications; the trunk posture of the elderly population in Southern Brazil using the Shadow Moire Technique; new physical therapy interventions for scoliosis; effects of load carriage on children with scoliosis; and the relationship of the pineal gland, melatonin and scoliosis.

Chapter I - Idiopathic scoliosis (IS) is a largely diffused disease in human population although its pathogenesis is still unknown. There is a relationship between IS phenotype and the patient age, since in the early stage the pathology shows a ratio of 50% between male and female childhood. During puberty the sex mainly involved into manifestation of disease is the female one, suggesting a sex-conditioned manifestation.

Chapter II - This presentation addresses the questions raised by the connections between idiopathic scoliosis, orthodontics and occlusion, as well as their therapeutic implications.

Idiopathic scoliosis makes its appearance before the end of the growth period, unassociated with other pathologies, which also differentiates them from scoliosis that are secondary to other problems such as malformations and neurological disorders. The etiology of idiopathic scoliosis is probably multifactorial, with components that are hormonal, connected with growth, with genetics, with metabolic disturbances of collagens and proteoglycanes, with neurological disturbances, and with biomechanical factors.

How should orthodontists deal with patients who suffer from idiopathic scoliosis? Does the malady exert a pernicious effect on the patient's occlusion? Will orthodontic treatment ameliorate or aggravate the patient's over-all health? These are the principal questions that must be answered when patients with scoliosis seek an orthodontic consultation.

Chapter III - Since 1970, the Moiré phenomenon has been employed as a method of clinical diagnosis in topographical analyses of the human body. This study aimed to evaluate the trunk posture of the elderly population in South Brazil using Shadow Moiré Technique (SMT). This is a cross-sectional, observational, exploratory and randomized study. SMT was applied to people over 60 years (n= 444; 331 women and 113 men) living in Porto Alegre-RS, Brazil. Lateral deviations of the thoracic spine, the alignment of scapula in the frontal and transverse planes, and the depth of torso were assessed. The data was presented as mean, standard deviation and percentiles (P5, P10, P25, P50, P75, P90, P95). Age and gender differences were tested using 2-way ANOVA followed by the Bonferroni post-hoc test whenever indicated ($p \leq 0.05$). The results for men showed a reduction in scapular alignment with progressive age, whereas this commenced in women only from 80 years of age. In relation to gender differences, men and women showed similarities in this variable for all ages. Thoracic kyphosis showed increases with age for men and women, and no statistical differences were found between genders. The age group 60-69 years showed statistical differences on right side gibosity ($p=0.002$), whilst for the left side, there were gender differences for the 60-69 years ($p=0.000$) and 70-79 years ($p=0.016$) age groups. There was no relationship between: the scapular alignment on frontal plane and angular spine variation on frontal plane; alignment between scapulas on transverse plane and angular spine variation on frontal plane of men and women. The results showed that SMT was useful for the evaluation of trunk deformities in the elderly.

Chapter IV - Scoliosis remains a common problem faced by orthopaedists and pediatricians worldwide. Current epidemiological studies place the prevalence of scoliosis at 3% in the general population. The commonest type of scoliosis is adolescent idiopathic scoliosis. To date, there have been many theories but no proven direct cause of idiopathic scoliosis. Genetics, central nervous factors, collagen, muscle and platelet defects, hormonal factors, as well as biomechanical factors seem to play a role in the development of this deformity.

Adolescents seldom complain of pain and often the first presentation to the orthopedist is following a referral from the primary care physician or a school screening program. The confirmation of scoliosis follows a radiograph showing at least 10 degrees of coronal deformity in the standing scoliosis x-ray. Back pain and pulmonary complications are rare in scoliosis except when the curve is severe. These problems are more pronounced in the infantile and juvenile scoliosis, often due to the rapid progression of the Cobb angle.

Chapter V - Introduction: Various non-invasive treatments have been used as interventions for mild to moderate scoliosis, those that are not severe enough to require surgery (40 degrees or less). While many of these have not shown to be efficacious, others have documented indicators of improvement. Despite the improvements obtained with conservative methods, individuals with scoliosis would benefit from more effective therapies. Purpose: To further study the effectiveness of the ATM2^{TM} for treatment of scoliosis. The ATM2^{TM} was previously shown to improve a scoliotic curve, in a published case study. Methods: Thirty-eight subjects were put on a therapy intervention using the ATM2^{TM} for eight to twenty sessions. Results: All subjects saw improvements in a variety of variables. Discussion: The ATM2^{TM} has shown to be a viable non-invasive intervention for the treatment of mild to moderate scoliosis.

Chapter VI - Scoliosis is a lateral spinal deformity. Despite extensive research, the etiology of scoliosis is still unclear. However, abnormal external loading is known to be one of the possible factors that may exacerbate the deformity. As load carriage is common for schoolchildren, it has been a concern whether an 'overweight' schoolbag would impose abnormal biomechanical and physiological stress on the spine. A series of investigations were conducted to compare the effects of backpack carriage on pulmonary function, standing posture and balance as well as gait performance in children with and without scoliosis. Pulmonary function and balance control in both standing and walking were found to be adversely affected by increased backpack weight. The effects of backpack carriage on children with and without scoliosis were similar. However, pulmonary function and stability control of children with scoliosis were consistently poorer than normal. The results of these studies showed that the limit of backpack weight recommended for normal children based on the changes in biomechanical and physiological measures might not be applicable for those with scoliosis. However, there is still a lack of evidence whether carrying backpack would accelerate curve progression in children with scoliosis. Further investigation is warranted to address this question.

Chapter VII - Over the past 25 years, chicken studies implicated experimental pinealectomy as acause of scoliosis. The nature of the scoliosis was demonstrated to be similar to that of human idiopathic scoliosis. Subsequent research involved a primate (Rhesus monkey) experimental pinealectomy model. Scoliosis was not induced by pinealectomy. In a recent Australian study, no causal link was established between pineal lesions and the development of idiopathic scoliosis. Melatonin is the only known hormone secreted by the pineal gland in humans. Previous research concluded that melatonin secretion was similar in those with idiopathic scoliosis and aged-matched controls. A recent Korean study concluded that permanent melatonin deficiency was not a causative factor in the aetiology of (AIS) adolescent idiopathic scoliosis. Over a period of 25 years, research involving the production of scoliosis following pinealectomy in small animal models has not been reproducible in the human model. The search for a scientifically sound human model to investigate the etiology of idiopathic scoliosis continues.

In: Scoliosis: Causes, Symptoms and Treatment   ISBN: 978-1-62081-007-1
Editors: A. Bessette et al.   © 2012 Nova Science Publishers, Inc.

Chapter I

Scoliosis: Causes, Genetics, Symptoms, and Treatment in a Southern Italy Population

*T. Esposito[1], B. Varriale[*1], G. F. DiMartino[2],
M. Chierchia[2], A. Gironi Carnevale[1] and D. Ronca[2]*
[1] Lab. of Molecular Genetics, Dept. of Experimental Medicine,
Faculty of Medicine and Surgery,
Second University of Naples, Naples, Italy
[2] Dept. of Orthopaedics and Traumatology,
Second University of Naples, Naples, Italy

Abstract

Idiopathic scoliosis (IS) is a largely diffused disease in human population although its pathogenesis is still unknown. There is a relationship between IS phenotype and the patient age, since in the early stage the pathology shows a ratio of 50% between male and female childhood. During puberty the sex mainly involved into manifestation of disease is the female one, suggesting a sex-conditioned manifestation.

---

[*] Corresponding author: Prof. B. Varriale, Lab. of Molecular Genetics, Dept. of Experimental Medicine, Faculty of Medicine and Surgery, Second University of Naples, Via Costantinopoli 16, 80138 Naples, Italy, e-mail: bruno.varriale@unina2.it.

Genetic inheritance of IS results still unclear although some evidences claim for a recessive multi-factorial inheritance. As far as it concerns the transmission of genetic traits involved in the IS phenotype, we have analysed 72 genealogical trees involving a total of 696 generations and 2416 individuals. For each transmission model we have evaluated using a not parametric analysis the number and percentage of compatible generations, number and total percentage of compatible individuals and number and average percentage of compatible individuals for each family. The results indicate a clear cut for an autosomic recessive trait (H=29.32, df3, p<0.000, Kruskal-Wallis test).There is, however, large agreement in considering the IS as a sex-conditioned disease, in terms of steroid content and their receptor activity. We have, recently, found a possible linkage between the estrogen content and the IS in a teenagers female population of southern of Italy. The 17β-estradiol, progesterone and testosterone contents in teens showing the IS phenotype is significantly lower with respect to unaffected girls ($P < 0.01$, <0.01 and <0.05, respectively). These data support the hypothesis of a reduced steroidogenesis in girls affected by IS. Because other authors have claimed for a linkage between the appearance of IS and some chromosomal region (chromosomes 6 and 10), we have undertaken a study having as target the possible linkage between the IS phenotype and polymorphisms for loci on both chromosomes 6 and 10.

The genetic loci we studied were 6p21.3 [17b-hydroxysteroid dehydrogenase (17b-HSD)], 6p21 [3b-hydroxysteroid dehydrogenase (3b-HSD)], 6q25.1 [estrogen receptor a (ERa)], 10q24.3 (17a-hydroxylase), 10q24.31 (21a-hydroxylase) and 10q24.32 (17,20 lyase). Polymorphisms in the coding regions in all gene studied have been found in girls affecting by IS, while the same polymorphisms have not been found in control girls. The 3b-HSD, the 17b-HSD, the 17a-hydroxylase, the 21a-hydroxylase and the 17,20 lyase are enzymes involved in the production of progesterone (3b-HSD), estradiol (17,20 lyase, 3b-HSD, 17b-HSD, 17a-hydroxylase) and testosterone (17,20 lyase, 3b-HSD, 17b-HSD, 17a-hydroxylase), respectively. It is conceivable that the polymorphisms that we have found may have a role in the relationship between the steroidogenetic enzymes (genotype) and the manifestation of IS phenotype, although more functional study on the effects of these polymorphisms could have on the enzyme activity. Among the ERa, we identified four polymorphisms in the exons encoding for the steroid binding domain and two other in the trans-activation domain that could have an effect on the receptor efficiency in binding the ligand in changing the Kd of the receptor protein. The overall data we have obtained, seem to indicate a linkage between the endocrine status and the IS phenotype in the affected girls.

History

The term *scoliosis* derives from the Greek word σκολιος, which means curvature. In Orthopaedics, it indicates a lateral curvature of the spine, which, normally, when viewed from the front or back, doesn't show any lateral deviation.

Hippocrates of Cos (460-377 B.C.) the first described in his book "De Articulationes" lateral curves of the spine and used the term *scoliosis* [1]. After him, Galen of Pergamo (129-216 A.D.) in "De Motu Musculorum" and Paul of Egina (625-690 A.D.) in his medical compendium in seven books (latin: *De re medica libri septem*), describe spine deformities and suggest various methods of treatment.

During the sixteenth century, Ambroise Paré (1517-1590), [2 which coined the word *orthopaedia*, described the deformity that we recognize today and suggested a treatment of scoliosis based on steel corset made by armourers. Later, Andry (1658-1742) [3] in his textbook of orthopaedics defined the deformity and postulated its pathogenesis. During the nineteenth century, many theories in the pathogenesis of scoliosis and many theories and therapies were proposed. At the end of this century, precise anatomic descriptions of the deformity from the autopsy were done and discovery of roentgen rays by Wilhelm Konrad Roentgen of Strassburg enhanced the knowledge of the factors involved in scoliosis.

The modern era in treatment of scoliosis began with Hibbs [4] and Forbes which the first performed the actual spinal fusion procedure for this disease, even dough the percentage of failure (pseudarthrosis) was too high. The pseudarthrosis rate has been lowered to an acceptable percentage by Cobb, Risser which paid close attention to cast correction, technique of fusion, and protection of the fusion until graft maturation. In 1946, Blount and Schmidt introduced a distraction brace, combined with lateral pressure pads, named Milwaukee brace. This brace was at first used only in the operative treatment of scoliosis [5-6]. Due to its success in curve correction, it was later used also in the nonoperative treatment of lesser curves. In 1960, Harrington instrumentation added internal stability to the fused spine and still today remains a milestone in the surgical treatment of the scoliotic spine [7].

In 1969, Dwyer A.F. of Australia obtained good results by a new method of correcting scoliotic curves by anterior disc excision combined with the insertion of special screws and compression of the vertebral bodies with a fixed cable [8]. Skeletal traction by *halo* was introduced by Nickel, Perry and

Garrett at Rancho Los Amigos, in Downey, California. Connected to a body cast, originally, the halo was used to provide spine distraction in paralytic spines. Later, the *halopelvic hoop* was developed by Dewald, in Chicago, to correct sever spine deformities [9]. Pierre Stagnara of Lyon, France, used the halo traction in a wheelchair with an overhead suspension.

Today, many techniques of correction, including various plaster jackets and braces, are proposed, but, unfortunately, in cases of severe spinal curvature, spinal fusion remains the only method of maintaining correction.

Classification

Scoliosis is defined as a lateral curve of the spine whit fixed rotation and permanent deformation of the vertebrae. More precisely, scoliosis is a deformity of the spine in all three space's planes: frontal plane (lateral curvature), horizontal plane (rotation of the vertebrae) and sagittal plane (deformity in lordosis or kyphosis). So, the true scoliosis must be distinguished from the scoliotic curve seen in the lumbar spine of a patient with inequality of leg length. In this case, when the leg length is corrected by a lift, or when the patient is in the sitting or supine position, the curve disappears; this curve has a normal mobility and never becomes structural. On the contrary, the true scoliotic curves are structural, characterized by distorted vertebrae with the body shifted toward the convex side of the thorax; moreover, the segment of spine with scoliotic curve shows a lack of normal flexibility (Figure 1).

When two curves in the same spine have the requirements of a structural curve, they are describes as a double structural curve. The structural curved can be also named primary or major curve (the original curve of the patient), whereas compensatory curve can be named secondary or minor curve. This concept of primary and secondary curves has been stressed by Cobb (1960). He pointed out that a primary curve is one produced by a deforming factor or force. A secondary curve is considered as the result of involuntary muscular action to centre the head on the pelvis as best as possible. Above or below a major curve exists a compensatory curve tending to maintain normal body alignment. It keeps the head over the pelvis and doesn't present fixed rotation nor permanent deformation of the vertebrae. However, in time (or as time goes by), the compensatory curve becomes structural, because the tissues develop fixation in this curved position. In this case, it can be difficult or impossible to know whether patient has one or two primary curves.

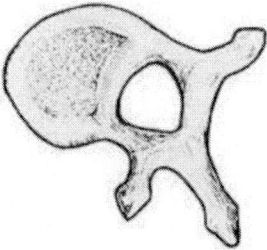

Figure 1. A distorted scoliotic vertebra with the body shifted toward the convex side of the thorax, the spinous process deviated to the concave side, and thick wide lamina on the concave aspect as compared with thinner elongated lamina on the convex side.

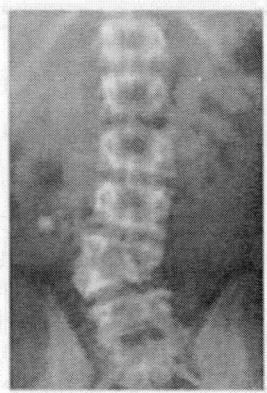

Figure 2. Congenital scoliosis due to lateral failure of formation (hemivertebra).

According to etiology, the scoliosis can be distinguished into two principal forms: congenital scoliosis (Figure 2) and acquired scoliosis [10]. The congenital scoliosis reflects anomalous development in utero and are due to congenital abnormalities, such as failure of formation (wedge, hemivertebrae), failure of segmentation (unilateral bar, fusion), myelomeningocele, meningocele, spinal dysraphism.

The acquired form must be divided into two groups: a) secondary scoliosis (or of known etiology), due to neuromuscular (poliomyelitis), myopathic, mesenchymal, metabolic, nutritional and endocrine disorders, traumatic causes (such as fracture or dislocation, deformities following thoracoplasty, neurofibromatosis, osteochondrodystrophies), Sheuermann's disease, Marfan's disease, Ehlers-Danlos disease, infection, tumor (cord tumors), syringomyelia and rheumatoid diseases); b) idiopathic scoliosis (of unknown etiology). The idiopathic scoliosis is the most common of all forms of scoliosis and accounts for 80-90 per cent of cases. In this form of scoliosis, the deformity consists of lateral deviation of the spine with rotation of the vertebrae. Frequently, a single major curve is observed, accompanied by one or two compensatory curves, that compensate for the spinal vertical alignment. It occurs during the growing years.

The idiopathic scoliosis are classified according to location, age at on set and magnitude. According to location, the curves are described in relation to the position of the end vertebrae and the apical vertebra. The end vertebra of the curvature is the most inclined and less rotated vertebra, corresponding to the last vertebra that is tilted into the concavity of the curvature; each curve shows a cranial and a caudal end vertebra; in other words, the end vertebra is the last vertebra that is tilting into the concavity of the curvature being measured. If there are parallel vertebrae at the end of a curve, the one farthest from the apex is the end vertebra. The apical vertebra is the most rotated, less inclined and most deviated vertebra from the vertical axis of the patient (Figure 3).

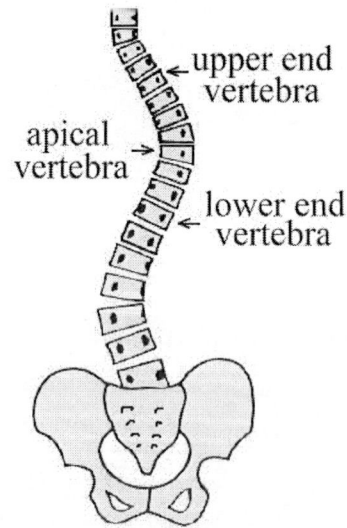

Figure 3. End vertebrae and apical vertebra are shown. See in the page for legend.

The idiopathic scoliosis have been classified by Ponseti and Friedman into five classes: *cervicothoracic*: the apical vertebra is T3, the upper end vertebra C7 or T1 and the lower end vertebra T4 or T5; *thoracic*: the apical vertebra is T8 or T9, the upper end vertebra at T6 or T7 and the lower end vertebra at T11 or T12; *thoracolumbar*: the apex is T11 or T12, the upper end vertebra at T6 or T7 and the lower end vertebra at L1 or L2; *lumbar*: the apex is L1 or L2, the upper end vertebra at L11 or L12 or T1 and the lower end vertebra at L4 or L5; *combined thoracic and lumbar*: the thoracic curve has its apex at T6 or T7, the lumbar curve has its apex at L2 [11]. We do not use the term dorsal interchangeably with thoracic, because anatomically all the vertebrae are dorsal with reference to the body. So, for the twelve dorsal vertebra we prefer the more anatomically correct term thoracic.

The degree of vertebral rotation is estimated by the position of the shadows of the pedicles and is classified into four grades [12]. Zero rotation: the pedicle shadows are equidistant from the sides of the vertebral bodies; Grade I rotation: the pedicle shadow on the convexity has moved from the edge of the vertebral body; Grade II rotation: rotation intermediate between Grade I and Grade III; Grade III: the pedicle shadow is close to the centre of the vertebral body; Grade IV: the pedicle shadow is past the centre of the vertebral body (Figure 4).

Once the curve and the end vertebrae have been identified, the magnitude and extent of each curve is determined by Cobb-Lippman technique of measurement [13]. The angle of the scoliotic curve is formed between two lines: a line is drawn at the upper end of the cranial end vertebra along the end-plate (or by marking the upper or lower edges of the pedicle shadows); a second line is drawn at the lower end of the caudal vertebra at the inferior end-plate of the body (or the lower end of the pedicle shadows). The angle is formed between two lines drawn at right angle to the two-end vertebral lines (Figure 5).

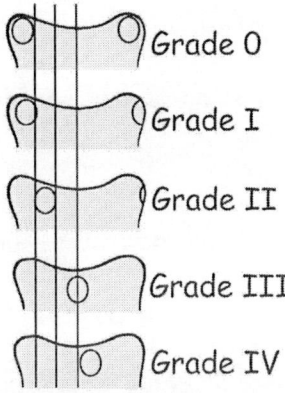

Figure 4. Schema of the 5 degrees of vertebral rotation.

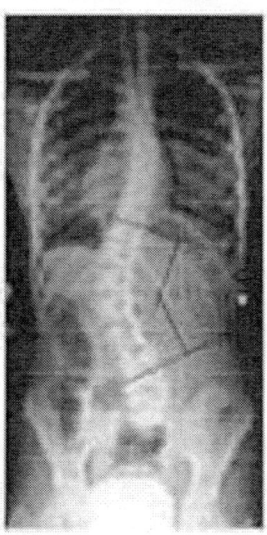

Figure 5. An idiopathic thoracolumbar scoliosis (T11-L4). Note the inclination and rotation of both end vertebrae and apical vertebra: no rotation (Grade 0) and maxima inclination of the end vertebrae, no inclination and maxima rotation (Grade II-III) of the apical vertebra. Note, also, the ossification of the iliac crest, that, in this case, is Risser stage 3.

In determining a patient's maturity three X-rays are used:

1. the radiograph of the left hand to evaluate the bone age compared to the standards radiographs found in the Greulich and Pyle Atlas [14].
2. the radiograph of the iliac crests to evaluate its ossification as described by Risser [15].

Normally, ossification starts at the anterior superior iliac spine and progresses posteriorly to the posterior superior iliac spine. Once complete ossification has occurred, fusion of the epiphysis with the ilium takes place, starting from posterior superior iliac spine and progressing anteriorly to the anterior superior iliac spine. Stage 0: no ossification of the iliac crest is present. Stage 1: ossification of 1/3 of the iliac crest has appeared; Stage 2: ossification of 2/3 of the iliac crest has appeared; Stage 3: ossification of 3/3 of the iliac crest has appeared; Stage 4: fusion of the 1/3 of the posterior iliac crest has taken place; Stage 5: fusion of the epiphysis has been completed (Figure 6).

3. the radiographs of the vertebral body to see grade of fusion of the vertebral ring apophyses, that lies at the upper and lower margins of the body overlying the cartilage growth plate and appear as a separate ossified area forming a complete ring. Fusion of the vertebral apophyses with vertebral body indicates the complete cessation of the spine growth.

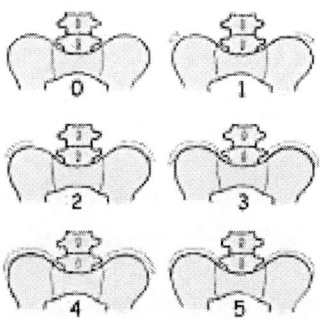

Figure 6. Schema of iliac crest ossification from 0 to stage 5, as described by Risser.

The age at onset is the age at which the deformity is first noted, which is not necessary the same as the time the curvature appears. Anyway, according to the age at onset, the idiopathic scoliosis is classified into 5 groups: 1) scoliosis of the new-born (from 1 month old to 12 months); 2) infantile (from 1 years old to 3 years); 3) juvenile from 4 years old to onset of puberty (according to Stagnara approach, we divide this stage into three subgroups: juvenile I: from 4 to 7 years old; juvenile II: from 8 to 10 years old ; juvenile III: from 11 years old to onset of puberty); 4) adolescent (from puberty to 18 years old); 5) adult (after 18 years old) [16].

It is known that scoliosis appearing later in adolescence usually has a better prognosis; in fact, the curvature ceases to progress about 1 year before complete ossification. A rapid increase in the curve on serial radiographs has a poor prognostic significance. Fortunately, only 5 to 10 per cent of idiopathic curves become severe enough to require surgical treatment [17]. In general, the earlier the onset, the worse the prognosis, because the idiopathic scoliosis develops during the growing years; so a scoliotic curve that appears during infantile age can increase much more than one appearing during adolescent age. Nevertheless, a large number of new-born scoliosis disappear spontaneously without treatment; these are the typical self-resolving idiopathic curves. This spontaneous resolution of the curve is noted less often in juvenile and adolescent curves.

Epidemiology

Idiopathic scoliosis (IS) is a largely diffused disease in human population although its pathogenesis is still unknown. There is a relationship between IS phenotype and the patient age, since in the early stage the pathology shows a ratio of 50% between male and female childhood. During puberty the sex mainly involved into manifestation of disease is the female one, suggesting a sex-conditioned manifestation.

Our study is derived from the examination of 4100 boys and girls from 6 schools. They ranged from ten to sixteen years old (average 12.0 years old). The first screening was made up of two young doctors, which eliminated children with normal spines. Those with deformities were then seen by one of us, and a radiographs where made for each student thought to have a spinal deformity. Deformities of the trunk other than scoliosis (Scheuermann's kyphosis, non-structural scoliosis associated with limb-length inequality, abnormalities of rib cage and spondylolisthesis) weren't considered. The films of those children with scoliosis were measured by Cobb's method and skeletal maturation was assessed by evaluating the development of iliac epiphysis using Risser's classification. The roentgenographic examinations showed that 224 students had a structural scoliosis, with an incidence of 5,4 per cent (Figure 7).

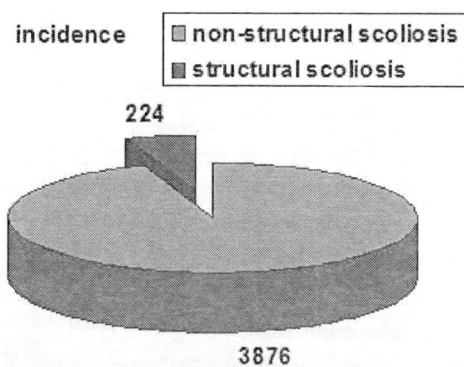

Figure 7. Diagram reporting the numbers of students with structural scoliosis end the normal ones.

The female-to-male ratio was 7.6:1.0 over-all (198 girls/26 boys) (Figure 8). Forty five per cent of the idiopathic curves were lumbar (101 curves, 91 females, 10 males); 21 per cent were thoracic (46 curves, 41 females, 5 males); 15 per cent were thoracolumbar (34 curves, 29 females, 5 males) and 19 per cent were double major (43 curves, 36 females, 7 males) (Figure 9, 10, 11, 12, 13).

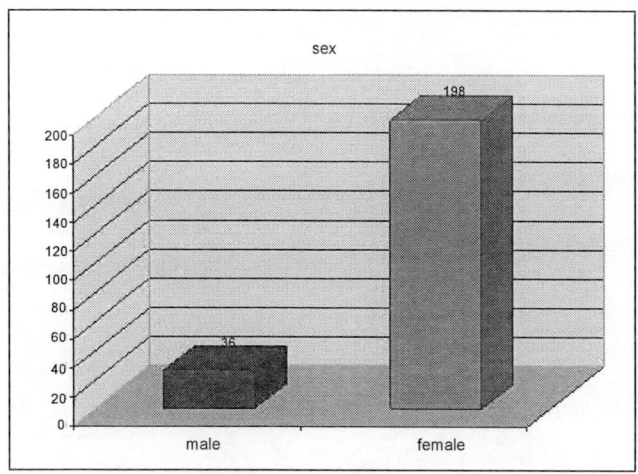

Figure 8. Distribution of IS between sexes.

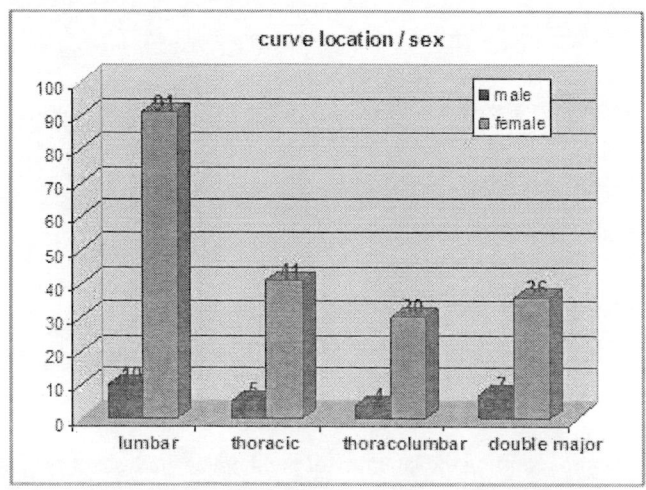

Figure 9. Diagram reporting the location of IS and the sex distribution.

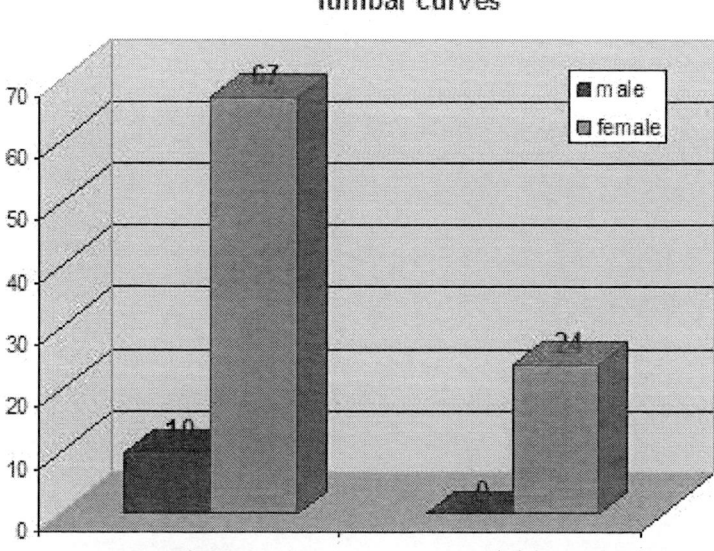

Figure 10. Diagram reporting the laterality of the lumbar curves and sex distribution.

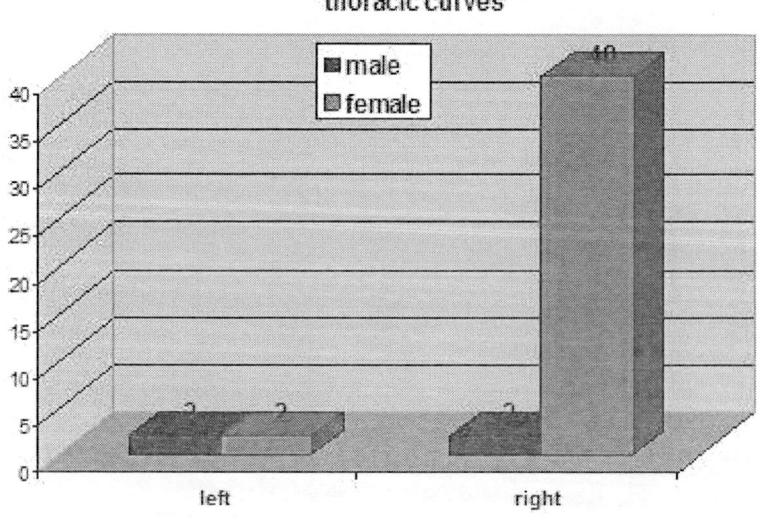

Figure 11. Diagram reporting the laterality of the thoracic curves and sex distribution.

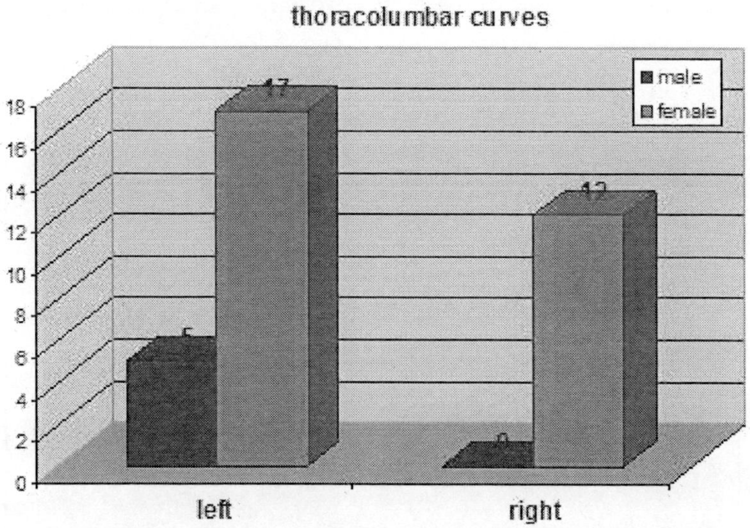

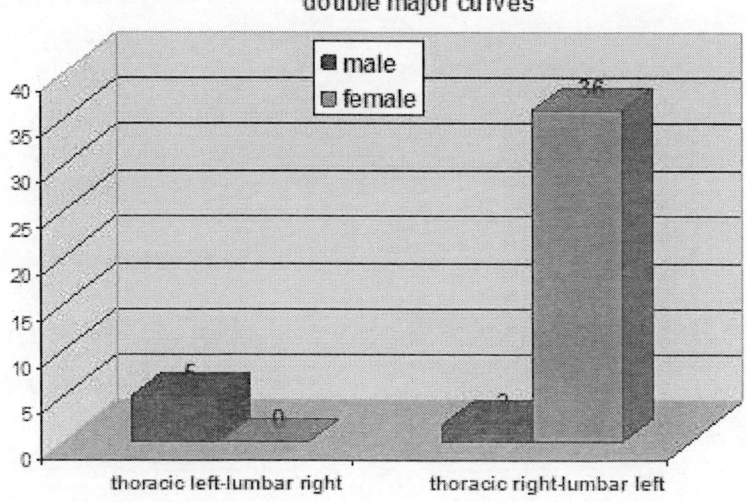

Figure 12. Diagram reporting the laterality of the thoracolumbar curves and sex distribution.

Figure 13. Diagram reporting the laterality of the double major curves and sex distribution.

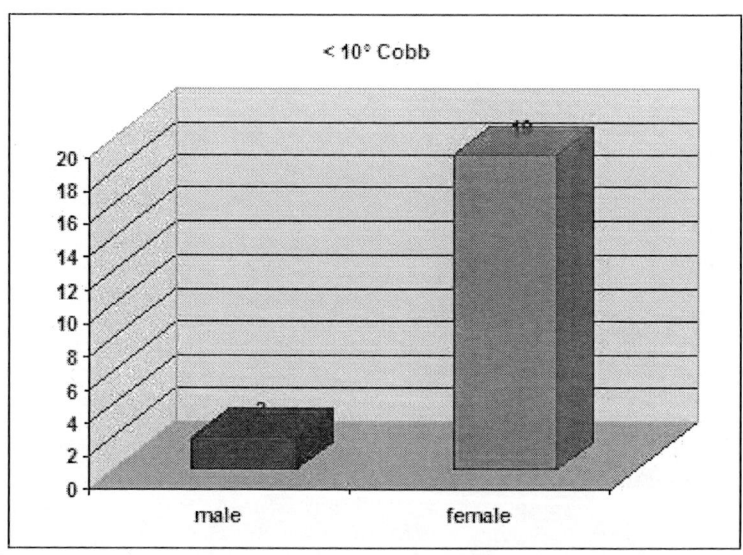

Figure 14. Diagram reporting the degree of curves lesser than 10° and sex distribution.

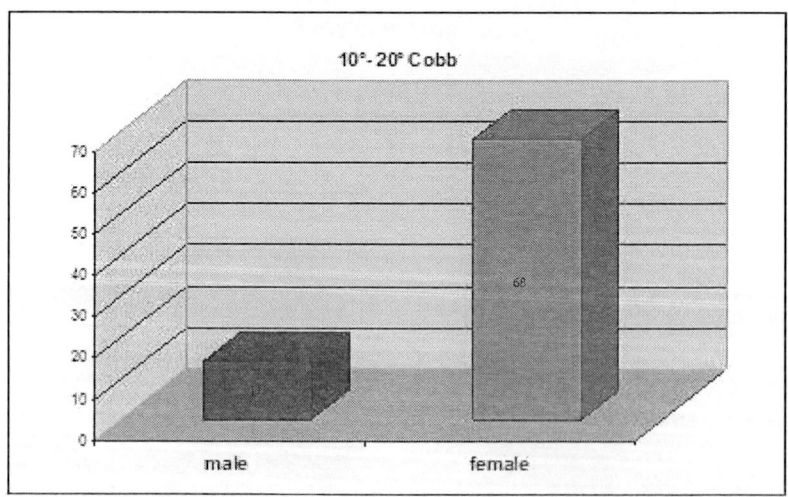

Figure 15. Diagram reporting the degree of curves between 10° and 20° and sex distribution.

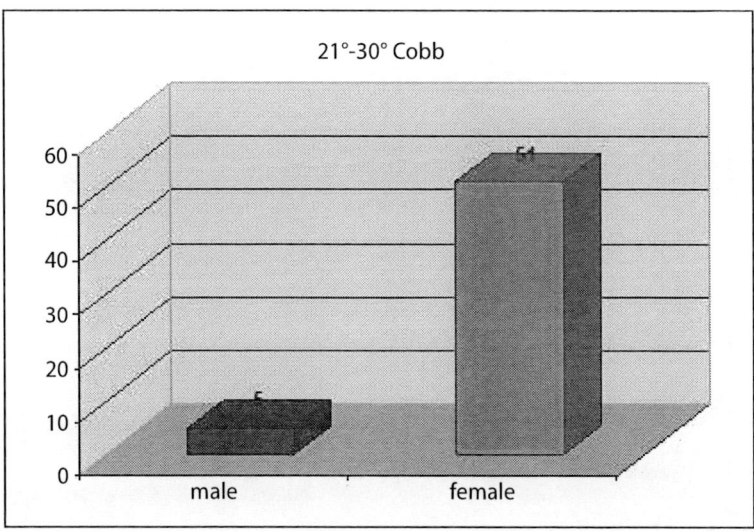

Figure 16. Diagram reporting the degree of curves between 21° and 30° and sex distribution.

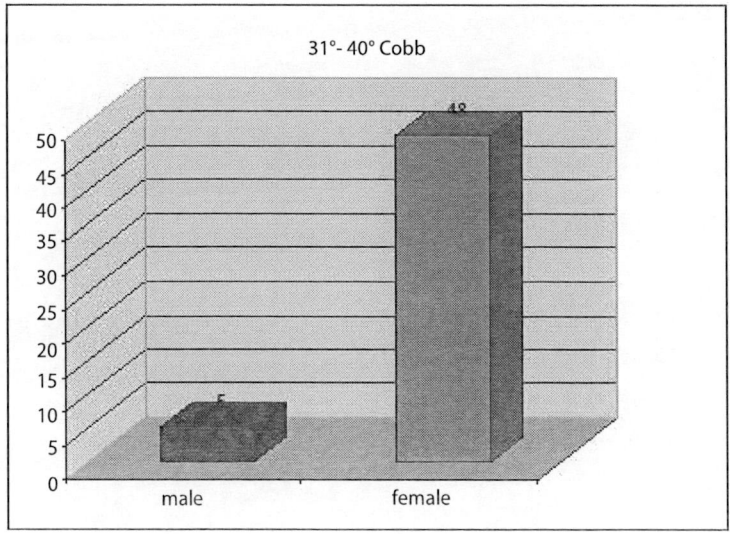

Figure 17. Diagram reporting the degree of curves between 31° and 40° and sex distribution.

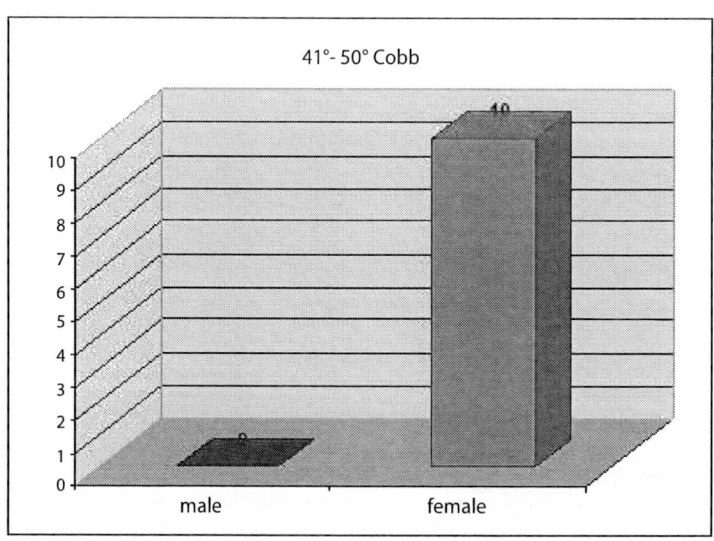

Figure 18. Diagram reporting the degree of curves between 41° and 50° and sex distribution

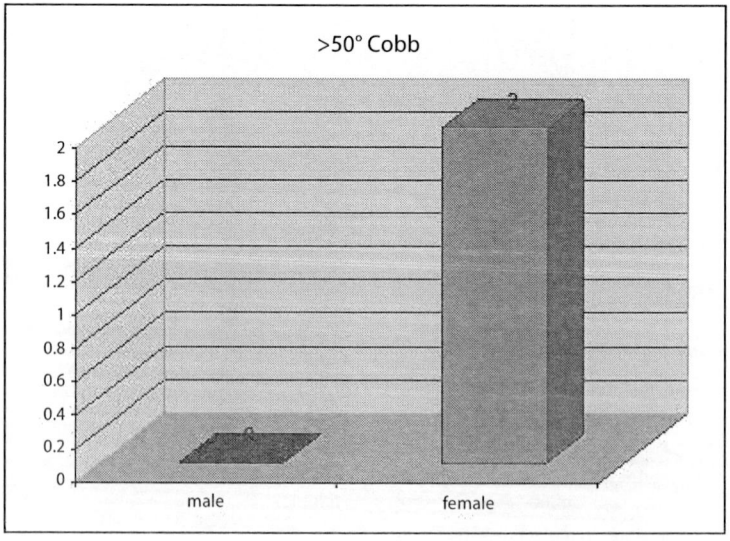

Figure 19. Diagram reporting the degree of curves over 50° and sex distribution.

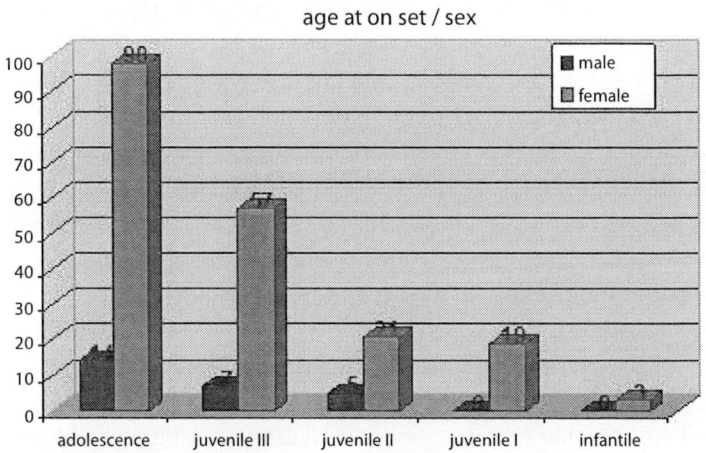

Figure 20. Diagram reporting the age at the onset and sex distribution.

The incidence of idiopathic scoliosis under 10 degrees was 0,5 per cent (21 curves, 19 females, 2 males); that of curves 10 and 20 degrees was 2 per cent (82 curves, 68 females, 14 males); for curves between 21 and 30 degrees was 13.6 per cent (56 curves, 51 females, 5 males); between 31 and 40 degrees 12.9 per cent (53 curves, 48 females, 5 males); between 41 and 50 degrees was 0.2 per cent (10 curves, all females); more than 50 degrees was 0.05 per cent (1 case, female) (Figure 14, 15, 16, 17, 18, 19). In our study, according to Brooks and Rogala [18-19], we included curves less than 10 degrees even tough is difficult to decide whether or not a curve les than 10 degrees is structural. Nevertheless, all these curves on repeated roentgenographic examinations showed to be structural.

With respect to the age at onset, the incidence of adolescence idiopathic scoliosis was 2,7 per cent (112 curves, 98 females, 14 males); juvenile III 1.5 per cent (64 curves, 57 females, 7 males); juvenile II 0.6 per cent (26 curves, 21 females, 5 males); juvenile I 0.4 per cent (19 curves, all females); infantile 0.07 per cent (3 curves, all females) (Figure 20).

Genetics of Idiopatic Scoliosis

The scientific advances of recent decades have made a significant increase in knowledge of the biological basis of many inherited diseases. In particular, studies on DNA have identified the molecular defects of many genetic diseases and the development of genetic tests that allow for accurate diagnosis in prenatal period.

And yet there are still many genetic diseases that are known in the clinical characteristics and mode of transmission, but not at molecular level. This implies that no specific genetic tests are available. There are also many genetic diseases with known mode of transmission and the molecular defect, and there is a genetic test, but for which there is still no effective therapy. Finally, there are complex genetic diseases defined, which are those most common in the general population, such as diabetes, cardiovascular disease or idiopathic scoliosis. These disorders are the result of multiple genes alteration, which, together with environmental factors, contribute to the development of the disease. For these specific genetic tests are not available, whereas it is important to trace the possible mode of transmission through the analysis of the pedigree. This is achieved performing a deep genetic counseling.

Genetic Counseling

Genetic counseling is a process through which information patients with a genetically determined disease, or their family, receive information concerning the characteristics of the disease, modes of transmission, the risk of recurrence and possible therapies, including reproductive options.

The precise diagnosis of the disease is prerequisite and necessary to perform genetic counseling. It can only be clinical or based on the assessment of specialists and on data derived from investigations, or may require the use of genetic testing. It can therefore sometimes be necessary to repeat earlier requests already made or remade.

Phases of Genetic Consulting in Individuals Affected by IS

Genetic counseling has been divided into several phases, which have required subsequent meetings between genetic consultant and proband family.

Collection of information has been done by personal and family history of the proband. This has been a pivotal moment, where have been gathered all the necessary information that aid us to shed light on the true origin of the genetic disease. Accurate information have been noted on the various members of the family, including those deceased, believed to have had the same disease. To this end it has been useful in addition to medical records and the various medical records, even photographs of deceased relatives.

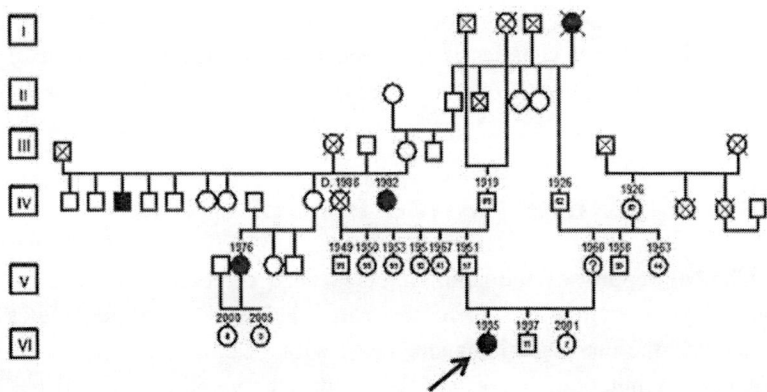

Figure 21. Typical familial tree of a girl affected by IS. It appears evident the autosomal recessive inheritance of the disease. The arrow indicate the proband.

Reconstruction of the family tree (pedigree, a graphic reconstruction that allows to collect genetic information of the family have been extended to at least three generations: the proband, parents, grandparents and relatives (Figure 21).

Specialist visits from genetics have been required to confirm or rule out other possible minimal signs of disease in the proband and his family.

Laboratory include genetic testing such as DNA analysis and/or chromosomes karyo-typing for those genetic diseases where the genetic defect is known, and instrumental examinations such as X-rays, CT scan etc.. In particular, the performance of genetic testing requires that those who submit to please review and approve an informed consent explaining the risks, limits and consequences of these tests.

The calculation of genetic risk give the possibility that a gene-based condition in the proband could happening again in other members of the same family. The risk calculation has been based on the assessment of mode of transmission of the disease, instrumental and laboratory data available and the position of the proband/s in the family. The genetic risk has been supplied in terms of probability or a percentage value.

Lastly there has been the communication time, where the specialist in medical genetics tells the proband/s or his family members the information obtained and the possible consequences. The advice haws been never to be directive and therefore should not influence the possible decisions of the proband/s or family.

The acquisition of data, communication of results and appropriate psychological support, in case of confirmation of genetic disease, stress as a specialist in medical genetics is the need to secure the cooperation of other professionals to achieve the goal of genetic counseling.

Inheritance Model for IS

Clinical reports of the familial occurrence of idiopathic scoliosis have appeared in the literature since the early 1930s. Population studies have documented the increased incidence of IS within families compared to that in the general population, suggesting that IS may be hereditary disorder [20, 21, 22]. Twin studies have consistently shown that monozygotic twins are more concordant for the condition than are dizygotic ones [23, 24]. Despite the evidence that this disese may have a major genetic component, the mode of inheritance is still unresolved. Studies have suggested both autosomal dominant and X-linked modes of inheritance [25, 26, 27]. Other studies have suggested that a multifactorial or polygenic mode on inheritance would explain the wide variability of scoliosis within and among families [22, 28]. Wynne-Davies [22] and Riseborough and Wynne-Davies [21] published two different series of studies with 2000 and 2869 individuals, respectively, suggesting either a dominant or multifactorial mode of inheritance. In 1972, Cowell *et al,* noting the paucity of male-to-male transmission in literature, selected 17 families (192 individuals) and reported a pattern of inheritance consistent with that of X-linked dominant inheritance [25]. Axenovich *et al* used complex segregation analysis to study 101 families (788 individuals) [29]. The results supported a genetic model; however, when the entire sample was considered, the best fitting genetic model was equivocal. When the authors excluded 27 families with probands with mild scoliosis, a Mendelian model with sex-dependent penetrances could not be rejected, suggesting that the disorder was the result of a single autosomal dominant locus.

Chan and coworkers have studied seven unrelated multiplex families of southern Chinese descent with AIS, consisting of 25 affected members. A genomewide scan >400 fluorescent microsatellite markers was performed. Multipoint linkage analysis by GENEHUNTER revealed significant linkage of the IS phenotype to the distal short arm of chromosome 19, with both a maximum multipoint LOD score and a nonparametric LOD score of 4.93. Two-point linkage analysis by MLINK gave a LOD score of 3.63 at D19S216. Further high-density mapping and informative recombinations defined the AID critical region in the vicinity of D19S216, flanked by D19S894, spanning 5.2 cM on the sex-averaged genetic map on chromosome 19p13.3 [30].

Informative recombinations observed in four of the families effectively narrowed the AIS critical region to around D19S216, between D19S894 and D19S1034, spanning 5.2 cM. This corresponds to a 1.9-Mbp region in the latest draft human genome sequence (Build 2.8). Within this region, there are about 71 possible gene sequences identified. Genes expressed in chondrocytes, osteoclasts, muscles, or tendon could be potential candidate genes for IS. Among these, the leucine-rich α-2-glycoprotein gene, which is similar to chondroadherin, expressed in chondrocytes, as well as the SH_3-domain GRB2-like 1 gene, which is similar to endophilin 2, expressed in osteoclasts, are two strong candidates. Sequencing of these genes to identify the molecular defect, as well as demonstrating segregation of the defect in all affected members of a family, would be necessary to establish their candidacy.

Four recent studies have reported possible relationship between marker loci and IS [22, 31,32,33]. Wise *et al* reported evidence for linkage on chromosome 6p, distal 10q, and 18q in a single extended family with IS in an affected-only analysis [31]. Salehi *et al* studied a single three-generation Italian family with IS and reported evidence of linkage to chromosome 17p11.2 [32]. Chan *et al* reported linkage to a 5.2 cM region on chromosome 19p13.3 in a group of 7 Chinese candidates and noted a second candidate region on chromosome 2 [22]. In a earlier analysis of the families in the current study, evidence of linkage was reported with markers on chromosome Xq23-26 in a subset of the families most likely to be X-linked dominant [33].

Model of Inheritance of IS

The study has been performed on 93 familial tree with a total number of 786 generations and 3416 individuals.

For each generation has been tested the concordance with all types of genetic inheritance: autosomal dominant, autosomal recessive, X-linked dominant and X-linked recessive.

The analysis of each inheritance model has been carried out having in mind the following parameters: number and percentage of compatible generations, number and total percentage of compatible individuals, number and mean percentage of individuals of each considered family.

The analysis have been performed using a non parametric test, the Kruskal-Wallis test [34].

a) Number and percentage of compatible generations

The model of inheritance autosomal recessive have shown to be those at most elevated compatibility since 364 generations (46.4%) well fit with this model of transmission. The other models have shown lesser compatibility with respect to the autosomal recessive one (17.1 X-linked dominant, 13.3 autosomal dominant and 9.9 X-linked recessive) (Figure 22).

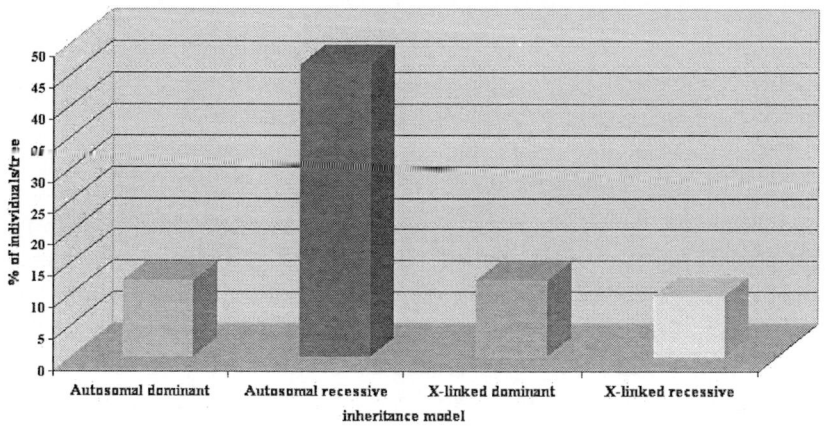

Figure 22. Analysis of the compatible generations with the various inheritance models. The analysis has been carried out using the non parametric analysis with the Kruskal-Wallis test. The autosomal recessive inheritance model is significantly higher than the other models.

b) Number and total percentage of compatible individuals

The analysis of this parameter also show the higher compatible values for the model autosomal recessive since 1581 individuals result compatible with this model of inheritance (46.3%). The other three models shown values greatly lower of compatible individuals (17.7% X-linked dominant, 11.5% autosomal recessive and 10.1% X-linked recessive).

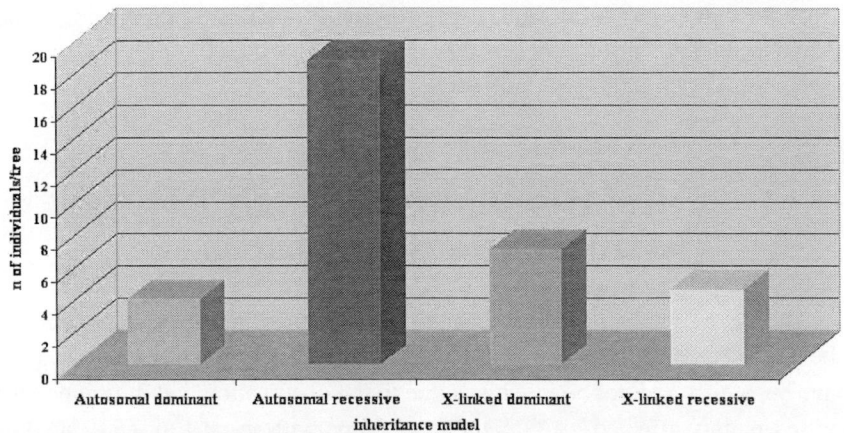

Figure 23. Analysis of the compatible individuals for each familial tree with the various inheritance models. The analysis has been carried out using the non parametric analysis with the Kruskal-Wallis test. The autosomal recessive inheritance model is significantly higher than the other models.

c) Number and mean percentage of compatible individuals for each family

This analysis have revealed the most elevated value of compatibility with the autosomal recessive model of inheritance showing a value of 18.9 individuals for each family. The other models shown values lesser than the autosomal recessive one (7.17 X-linked dominant, 4.67 autosomal recessive and 4.08 X-linked recessive) (Figure 23).

It is worth to note that the values of the analyzed family have not satisfied Levene's test [35] indicating that there is unequal variance across generations. As a consequence a non-parametric analysis has been performed. As a matter of fact, a series of non-parametric ANOVAs by Kruskal–Wallis test confirmed significant differences among autosomal recessive model, with respect to the other models, showing higher values of hereditability (H=29.32, df3, p<0.000)

In considering the mean percentage of compatible individuals for each family the analysis performed suggests once again the higher value of compatibility with autosomal recessive model having a value of 46.6% vs the values of the other models of transmission (17.2% X-linked dominant, 12.2% autosomal dominant and 9.7% X-linked recessive).

Since the analysis of the 93 family have not satisfied Levene's test indicating that there is unequal variance, a non-parametric analysis was performed. As a matter of fact, a series of non-parametric ANOVAs by

Kruskal–Wallis test confirmed significant differences among autosomal recessive model, with respect to the other models, showing higher values of hereditability (H=34.85, df3, p<0.000).

Relationship between IS and Endocrine Status

Before to focus on this aspect of the picture that characterize the IS phenotype it is important to stress the concept that the subject of our study have been girls and not boys. This is due to the observation that during puberty the sex mainly affected by IS is the female one with respect to male one. Our population sample show a ratio female/male of 7.6:1.0.

The structural changes that occur in IS, concerns directly the osseous part of spine, its ligamentous and capsular apparatus as well as muscular system. In this respect, bone development, occurring during puberty in human is a critical period for a well development of bone in general and spine in particular. On the other hand, the role of steroid hormones in the development and maintenance of bone is a well-established phenomenon. It is traditionally accepted the point of view that estrogens and androgens were the main sex steroids influencing bone maturation and maintenance in women and men, respectively. Studies reported that serum 17 β-estradiol well correlated with bone mass density although also T has some effects [36, 37, 38, 39, 40, 41, 42, 43, 44, 45, 46]. It has been shown that serum 17β-estradiol is important in the increase in bone mass during the puberty [47]. This claims for a central role of estrogen with respect to skeletal metabolism. In fact, in patients with aromatase deficiency 17β-estradiol levels lesser than 20 pg/ml are required to complete bone maturation and mineralization [48, 49, 50, 51].

In the population of female teenagers we have studied the focus was the endocrine status of teenagers affected by IS. Low levels of 17β-estradiol, testosterone and progesterone, have been found only in girls affected by IS, while normal values have been found in the control unaffected girls (Figure 24, 25, 26)[52]. This finding well correlate with international reports on the role of steroid on bone development during the puberty.

However the low blood concentrations of 17β-estradiol, testosterone and progesterone may belongs either to low level of steroid production by follicular cells or to low levels of the enzymes involved in steroid conversion.

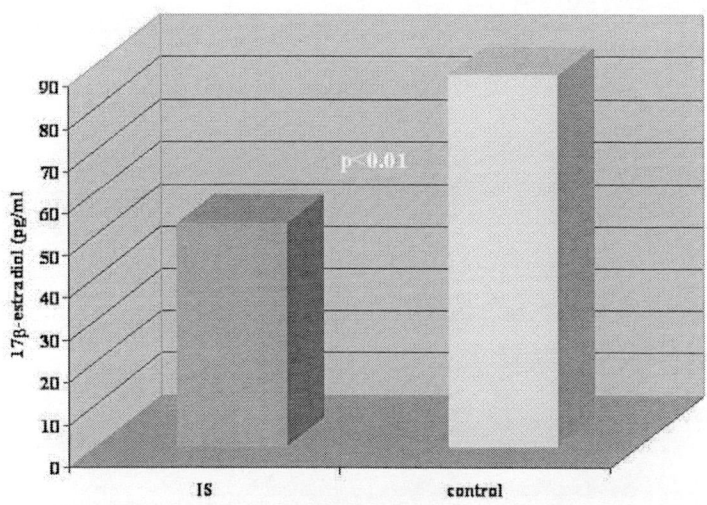

Figure 24. 17 β-estradiol content in blood samples from teenagers with IS phenotype (IS) and in teenagers not showing IS (control). Each blood sample was collected during the ovulatory phase. In IS teenagers the 17β-estradiol content was significantly ($p < 0.01$) lower than no IS teenagers (control).

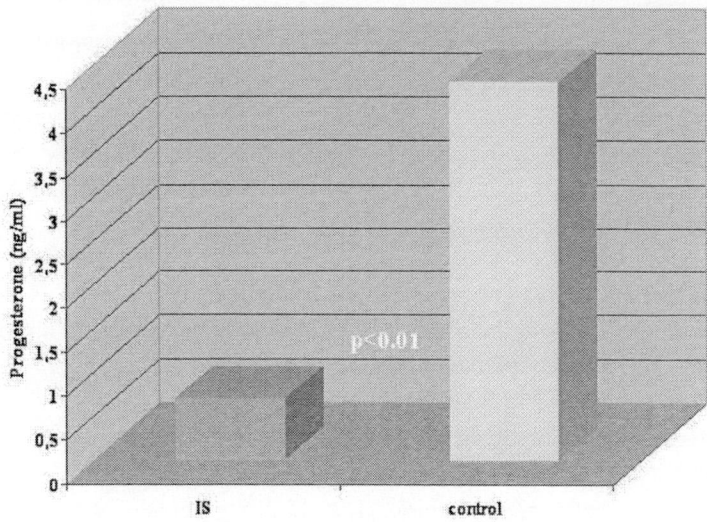

Figure 25. Progesterone content in blood samples from teenagers with IS phenotype (IS) and in teenagers not showing IS (control). Each blood sample was collected during the ovulatory phase. In IS teenagers the progesterone content was significantly ($p < 0.01$) lower than no IS teenagers (control).

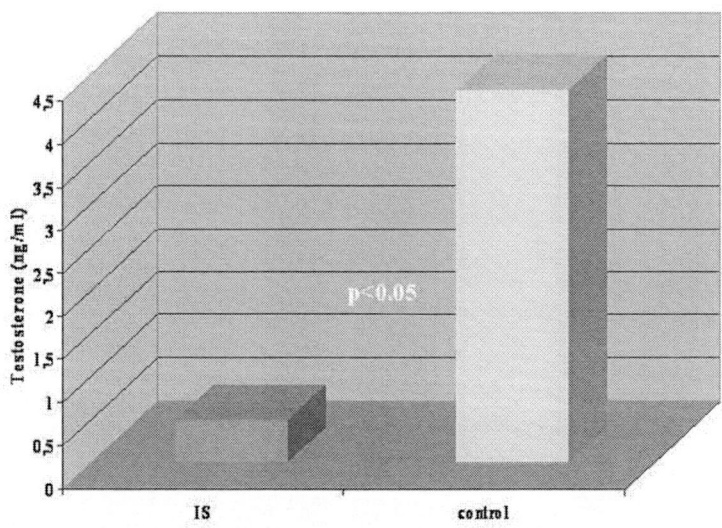

Figure 26. Testosterone content in blood samples from teenagers with IS phenotype (IS) and in teenagers not showing IS (control). Each blood sample was collected during the ovulatory phase. In IS teenagers the testosterone content was significantly ($p < 0.01$) lower than no IS teenagers (control).

It is noteworthy that during genetic coucelling the majority of the affected girls referred the use of contraceptive adjuvant since frequently their ovarian cycle was irregular. This fact let us to suppose that the lower endocrine status, of girls affected by IS, with respect to not IS girls, is probably due to a reduced production of steroids than to a reduced conversion. This finding let us to hypothesize that in teenagers, affected by IS, a reduced levels of steroidogenesis occur.

In this respect, linkage studies on polymorphisms in the enzymes involved into steroidogenesis and the occurrence of IS would be extremely informative. In our teens population affected by IS we have found a series of point mutation in the coding region of 17,20 lyase (Figure 27, 28).

This enzyme is involved into conversion of dehydro-epiandrosterone to androstendiol. Androstendiol is successively converted into testosterone by 3β-hydroxy steroid dehydrogenase. The 17,20 lyase is also involved into conversion of 17α-hydroxy progesterone into androstenedione being the latter converted into testosterone by the 17β-hydroxy steroid dehydrogenase. This observations well correlate with a reduced levels of steroidogenesis in girls affected by IS, since in unaffected girls a wild-type 17,20 lyase occurs and a normal stroidogenesis has been observed.

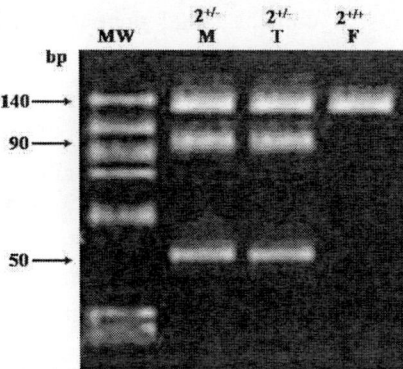

Figure 27. Analysis of FRLP generated by digestion with HhaI enzyme of amplified products of the exon 2 belonging form 17/20 lyase gene. F = father; T = teenager; M=mother. Number above the tested samples indicate their genetic status (+/+ wild type) (+/- heterozygous).

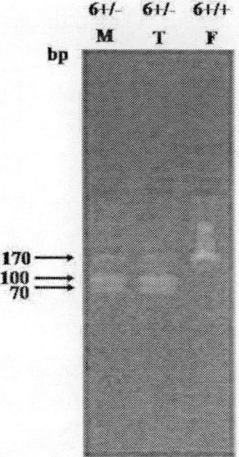

Figure 28. Analysis of FRLP generated by digestion with MspjI enzyme of amplified products of the exon 6 belonging form 17/20 lyase gene. F = father; T = teenager; M=mother. Number above the tested samples indicate their genetic status (+/+ wild type) (+/- heterozygous).

Estrogen Receptor Polymorphism and IS

The cortical bone size is, at least partly, due to sex steroid exposure during sexual maturation. In mice, it has been demonstrated that androgen receptor

(AR) activation results in cortical radial bone expansion [53], since male AR−/− mice have reduced cortical bone development. This also claims, for a role of T in bone development. In addition, male ERα−/− but not ERβ−/− mice show reduced cortical radial bone growth during sexual maturation. These results indicate that ERα but not ERβ activation is also important for a normal cortical radial bone growth [12]. Similarly as seen for cortical bone, both AR and ERα but not ERβ activation regulates trabecular bone mass in mice [32, 51, 53]. Studies on the effect of ER activation on trabecular bone have been performed in order to better understand which ER is mainly involved in bone development. In these studies, orchidectomized wild type (WT) and ER-inactivated mice were treated with the non-aromatizable androgen dihydrotestosterone (DHT), 17β-estradiol, or vehicle. Both ERα and AR but not ERβ activation preserved the amount of trabecular bone. ERα activation resulted both in a preserved thickness and number of trabeculae. ERα is the principal ER for the regulation of both trabecular and cortical bone in female mice [54, 55, 56, 57, 58]. Thus, the activation of ERα, may have a central role in the bone homeostasis.

The study on our teens population affected by IS have shown polymorphic sequences in the exons 5–8 of the ERα (Figure 29, 30, 31, 32).

It is noteworthy that the exons 5,6 and 7 encode for the steroid binding domain of ERα and each point mutation has the effect to change the amino-acid sequence of the domain itself.

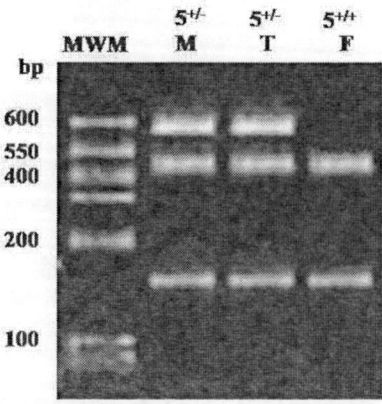

Figure 29. Analysis of FRLP generated by digestion with XbaI enzyme of amplified products of the exon 5 belonging form ERα gene. F = father; T = teenager; M=mother. Number above the tested samples indicate their genetic status (+/+ wild type) (+/− heterozygous).

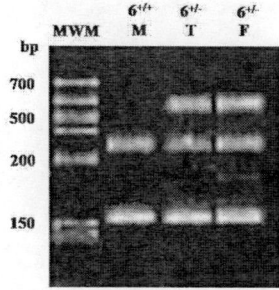

Figure 30. Analysis of FRLP generated by digestion with Pst1 enzyme of amplified products of the exon 6 belonging form ERα gene. F = father; T = teenager; M=mother. Number above the tested samples indicate their genetic status (+/+ wild type) (+/- heterozygous).

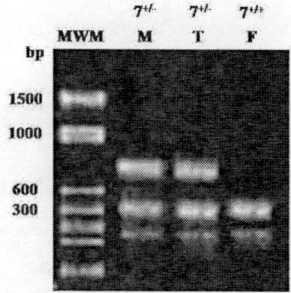

Figure 31. Analysis of FRLP generated by digestion with StuI enzyme of amplified products of the exon 7 belonging form ERα gene. F = father; T = teenager; M=mother. Number above the tested samples indicate their genetic status (+/+ wild type) (+/- heterozygous).

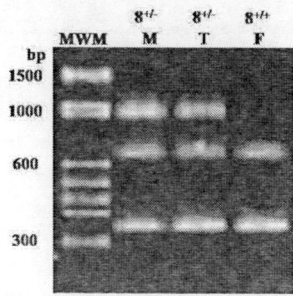

Figure 32. Analysis of FRLP generated by digestion with MseI enzyme of amplified products of the exon 8 belonging form ERα gene. F = father; T = teenager; M=mother. Number above the tested samples indicate their genetic status (+/+ wild type) (+/- heterozygous).

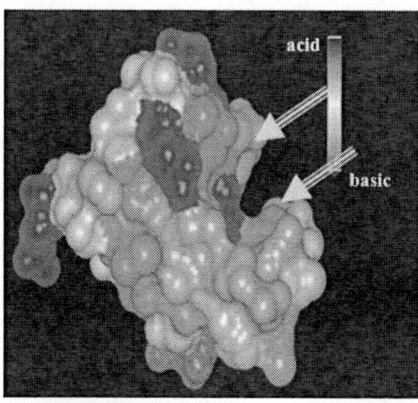

Figure 33. Spatial structure of the human ERα protein. The arrows indicate the point of amino acids substitution in the steroid binding pocket. These substitution have the effect to change the electric properties of the pocket itself, leading to a probably reduced affinity of the ligand with protein.

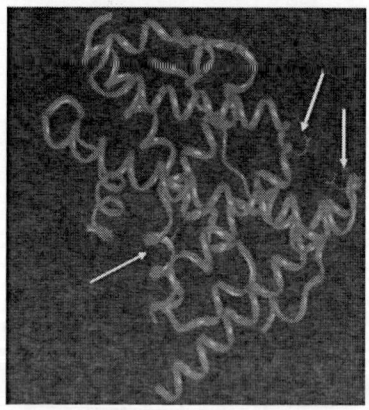

Figure 34. Spatial structure of the human ERα protein. The arrows indicate the point of amino acids substitution. These substitution are in the α-helix motifs of the proteins and being mainly substitutions with a change in the electrical properties of the protein may have the effect to reduce the dissociation constant of the protein with respect to the binding with steroid.

In the exon 5 the Leu^{379} is substituted by Glu. Thus a non-polar amino-acid is substituted by a basic one. In the exon 6, the Glu^{441} is substituted by Gln. Thus a basic amino-acid is substituted by a polar one. In the exon 7 the Leu^{495} is substituted by Met with not relevant changes in amino-acid characteristics (Figure 33, 34).

To our knowledge, no report of such mutations has been reported in the international literature, despite numerous mutation of the ERα has been found or experimentally induced [59]. Furthermore, these point mutations, are not present in the control girls, and in the IS girls we never found more than one mutation. It is conceivable that the above mutation could have an effect on the reduction of the affinity of the ligand pocket with steroid, that in turn could modify the Kd of steroid/receptor binding.

On the other hand, the reduced levels of steroids in teenagers with IS are probably *per se* the mastermind in the regulation of the homeostasis of estrogen/ERα function. However, it is also conceivable that both the reduced stroidogenesis and ERα mutations, could be implied in IS phenotype.

Clinical Evaluation

Commonly, scoliosis is noticed during summer months when the children are at the beach and their backs are exposed. Unequal shoulder height, unilateral prominence of the hip, posterior protrusion of a scapula or unilateral prominence of the breast are the most common observations. Frequently, the scoliosis is accompanied by few symptoms, among which an occasional feeling of tiredness in the lumbar area; even thought, in case of severe scoliosis shortness of breath may occur due to consequent deformity of the chest. On the contrary, whit advancing age, can arise the pain of osteoarthritis, radiculitis or the pain of impingement of the ribs on the iliac crests.

Physical examination has done with child completely disrobed to define the shoulder heights, prominence of a flank and/or of posterior ribs with overlying scapula. The chest is inspected and the state if maturity of the child is noted in terms of breast development in girls and pubic hair development in both sexes. The patient is principally examined from the back to evaluate the spine deformity (Figure 35, 36).

Trunk alignment must be noticed by use of a plumb line to demonstrate if the body attempts to place the skull over middle of the sacrum. This measure is of important prognostic significance indicating a possible quick progression of the deformity when this alignment has not reached; that means that spine is not in balance. It can be determined dropping a plumb line from the occiput to the natal cleft and measuring in centimetres the distance of this line to the right or left Figure 37).

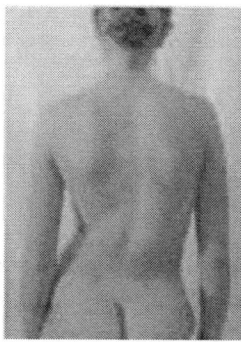

Figure 35. A typical right thoracic curve is shown. Note the decreased distance between the right arm and the thorax that is shifted to the right. The left iliac crest is just apparently higher because of the shift of the thorax with fullness on the right and elimination of the waistline.

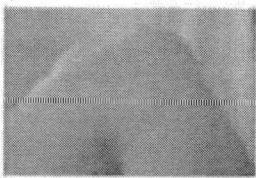

Figure 36. Forward bending test. The patient stands with feet together and knees straight and bends forward at the waist. The hands are held together, fingers and palms opposed. Note the presence of a right thoracic prominence, that is measured in centimetres.

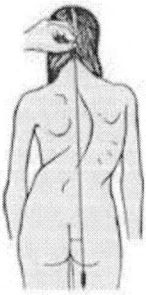

Figure 37. Plumbline dropped from the prominent vertebra C7 to the gluteal cleft to measure the decompensation of the upper torax over the pelvis. The distance from the vertical plumbline to the gluteal cleft is measured in centimetres.

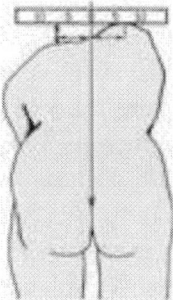

Figure 38. Measurement of the prominence. The level, made horizontal, is positioned with zero mark over the palpable spinous process in the area of maximal prominence: the distance to the apex of the deformity is noted; the perpendicular distance from the level to the valley is measured at the same distance from the midline.

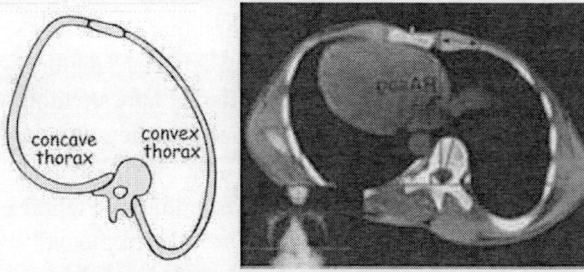

Figure 39. The deformity of scoliosis results in the rotation of the vertebral bodies into the convex thorax. With rotation of the attached ribs, the convex thorax becomes significantly diminished, and although the concave thorax appears enlarged, the net effect is a decrease in overall volume.

    The rib hump measurement to know the thoracic cage deformity is useful to know. With patient flexed forward 90 degrees, it is recorded measuring, in millimetres, the difference between the convex rib hump and concave rib depression. When more than one prominence is present, each one is evaluated in a similar manner, noting the side and the site of the prominence (thoracic, lumbar or thoracolumbar). In scoliosis, due to distorsion and rotational deformity of the spine, an anterior prominence is present on the side opposite the posterior rib prominence (Figure 38).

    The scoliotic deformity is characterized by distorted vertebrae with the body shifted toward the convex side of the thorax, the spinous process deviated to the concave side, thick wide laminae on the concave aspect and tin elongated laminae on the convex side (Figure 39). The convex side of the thorax is markedly decreased in size by an acutely angular deformity of the rib with a correspondingly opposite change on the concave side, resulting in a significant decrease in the entire volume of the thorax. These changes result in the alterations of vital capacity that are usually seen with thoracic scoliosis. In fact, patients with severe curvature show markedly increased disability and shortened life expectancy [60]. There is a tendency for thoracic scoliosis to have a diminished sagittal chest diameter, which is part of the cosmetic deformity and may contribute to restrictive lung disease. The oxygen tension is generally reduced, carbon dioxide tension increased, and oxygen saturation diminished; vital capacity, residual volume, and total ling capacity are significantly reduced in these severe cases.

The most deforming curves originate early in the life. The structural changes in the vertebrae responsible for scoliosis is principally due to the development of a wedge-like deformity of the vertebral body. Accompanying this, are the rotational defects in the involved vertebrae which appear as the lateral deviation develops. It is generally assumed that rotation is secondary to lateral deviation [61]. No constant ratio exists between lateral deviation and rotation of the vertebral bodies; the rotational defect appears more resistant to correction. Rotary displacement can be recognized on the spine radiographs by lateral displacement of the spinous process and by the asymmetry of the shadows of the pedicles in relation to the corresponding vertebral bodies. The pedicles on the convex side of the curvature are placed medially away from the lateral borders of the bodies on that side, while the pedicles on the concave side become less distinct and in same severe cases disappear from view completely. The neural arches of the rotated vertebrae likewise becomes deformed, and the articular facets on the concave side are thrown out of alignment with those on the convex side, with consequent locking of vertebrae in their rotated position.

Radiographic Evaluation

The radiographic evaluation of the deformity is the most valuable diagnosis tool available to the orthopaedic surgeon. It allows to evaluate the curvatures in terms of site, magnitude, flexibility and patient maturity. The spine radiographs are all viewed as if viewing the patient from the back; that is, the right side of the patient is viewed on the right side of the radiographs.

For proper evaluation of a scoliotic curve a complete radiograph series it's essential to have. This series includes: 1) an erect antero-posterior and lateral view of the entire spine from the iliac crest up to the cervical region, preferably on a 36-inch cassette, that provide both angular scoliosis deformity and information with regard to the further growth potential of the vertebrae by Risser method; 2) an antero-posterior view of the left hand and wrist for comparison with the Atlas of Gruelich and Pyle, in order to establish bone age, in the patient under age 20; 3) lateral side bending films to determine flexibility of the scoliotic curve. The antero-posterior view of the entire spine should be carried out every six months.

Treatment

In the treatment of scoliosis there is an axiom *"Do not allow progression to occur"* [62]. In fact, the vertebral deformity can only increase and the patients treated early do well not only in our experience. In general, the treatment of scoliosis depend on the age of the patient, on the location and magnitude of the primary curve. According to magnitude, we classify the scoliotic curve into three groups: 1) under 25°-30°; 2) from 25°-30° to 45°-50°; 3) over 45°-50°. For the group 1, we adopt only physical exercises just to improve bad posture and pulmonary function, because none exercise alone will not correct a progressive curve nor affect the natural history of the curvature. This approach is carried out in juvenile and adolescent scoliosis; in case of infantile scoliosis, even thought the curve measures less of 25 degrees, is necessary to use a brace, because the infantile scoliosis is a different entity from the juvenile and adolescent type and often continues to progress throughout juvenile and adolescent years.

Non Operative Treatment

Recent studies of the natural history of untreated scoliosis indicate that many idiopathic scoliosis of less 30° are non progressive [63] particularly in postpuberal children or children with advanced skeletal maturity. This fact focuses attention on current indications for brace treatment. We think that, unless the patient is nearly skeletal mature, is necessary to treat all curves in excess of 30° on the assumption that left untreated most curves of more 30° will progress with remaining growth.

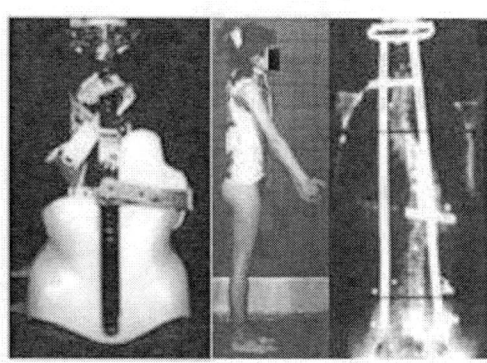

Figure 40. Front and lateral view of the Milwaukee brace. AP radiographs of an idiopathic infantile thoracolumbar scoliosis.

For the scoliosis of second group, nonoperative treatment includes the use of different type of brace, in relation to the age and the location of the curve. Brace treatment of scoliosis remains the only widely accepted and documented affective non operative treatment of progressive idiopathic scoliosis. In infantile and juvenile I and II scoliosis, we use the Milwaukee brace developed in 1945 by Blount and Schmidt [64].

As it is currently used, it emphasizes active and passive correction and derotation with lateral direct force (Figure 40).

It consists of a molded, well fitting pelvic section, two posterior uprights and a single anterior upright which connect the pelvic section to the neck ring. The neck ring has a throat mould and two occipital pads. Well fitted lateral pads are connected to the uprights to correct the specific deformity. From the beginning, this brace has proved to be the first device that can effectively control the scoliosis deformity. As stressed by Blount, the correction by the Milwaukee brace provides two important aspects: the distraction component and the active correction by the patient itself. His mechanism of correction is to relieve pressure on the concave side of the vertebral growth plate. The physical exercises are an important adjunct to treatment with brace, improving significantly the final result. According to some reports, the median final correction performed by the Milwaukee brace is 20 to 25% [65], with much more success in lumbar and thoracolumbar curves [66]. Treatment with Milwaukee brace requires the service of the orthopaedic surgeon, an orthotist, and a physiotherapist. The brace is worn for 23 hours a day, also at night, because of tendency of children to assume a position of scoliotic deformity during sleep. To be effective, this brace, as any other brace, must be carefully supervised and combined with exercises. Few restrictions are imposed; in fact, the patient is allowed to participate fully in all activities. When radiographs indicate the complete growth of the vertebrae and removal of the brace for increasing periods demonstrates retention of the correction, the brace is gradually removed.

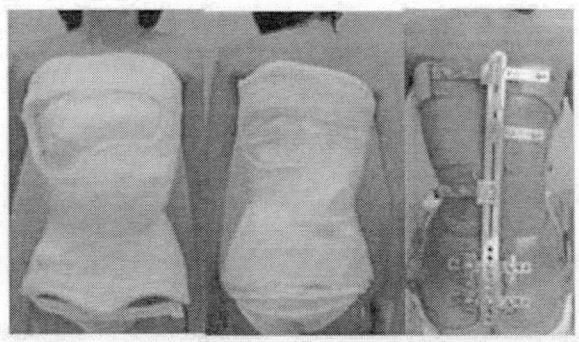

Figure 41. Front and back view of E.D.F. cast and back view of a plastic brace in an idiopathic juvenile III thoracic right scoliosis.

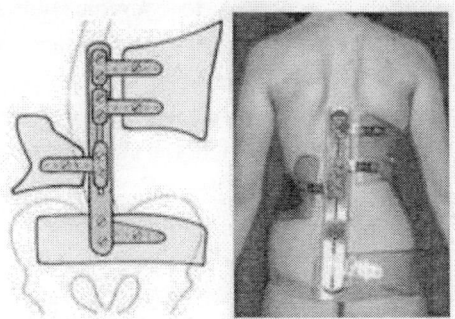

Figure 42. Back view of the "three-point brace" in an idiopathic juvenile III lumbar left scoliosis.

In juvenile II and III scoliosis and in adolescent scoliosis, we use the treatment carried out by Cotrel in 1954 [67] that includes a series of three E.D.F. (elongation, derotation, flexion) casts, changed every 45 days. After this period, the child is placed in a plastic corset till to complete growth of the vertebrae (Figure 41). A coordinate exercise program is useful in these patients as a prophylaxis against the stiffness and weakness induced by brace wear.

In this group, when the curve is located at lumbar site, we use the "three-point brace" developed in Lyon, France, in 1971, by Michel and Allègre [68]. This is a short plastic brace that doesn't require a preliminary cast for initial correction of deformity. Because of its small dimension, there is a good compliance both from parents and patients for this corset. As Milwaukee brace, the 3-point brace emphasizes an active and passive correction with lateral direct force (Figure 42). This corset operates on two principles: the first one is the three-point principle, the three points being the pelvic pad, the lumbar pad and the thoracic pad over the convexity of the lumbar curve. The second principle of correction is done by the wedge-shape of the lumbar pad, which, like a "wedge", has the role of opening the iliac-lumbar angle, essential to correct the scoliotic curve. As usual, a physical therapy program is necessary to minimize trunk weakness or stiffness that the patients may have from using the brace. Exercises to enhance active correction in the brace are recommended.

The same indications has the Boston brace, introduced in 1971 by Hall and Miller [69]. The Boston bracing system, widespread used, consists of a prefabricated thoracolumbar pelvic module that makes use of areas of relief opposite pressure areas and emphasizes lumbar flexion. A coordinated physical therapy program is necessary to overcome the relative hip flexion contracture experienced by many patients when they are placed in the position of lumbar flexion demanded by the brace.

As 3-point brace, use of Boston brace appears significantly to improve the course of scoliotic curves between 30 and 45° in immature individuals [70].

Operative Treatment

In cases where stable correction cannot be achieved, operative treatment must be considered without delay to avoid that many patients can been allowed to progress to a large and more rigid curve. The operation consists in the surgical posterior bilateral fusion of the spine achieved by facet joint destruction, bony decortication, autogenous bone grafting and adequate immobilization. With Harrington instrumentation, the correction is achieved by distraction device, which is inserted superiorly into the articular facets or lamina and inferiorly into the superior surface of the lamina (Figure 43) [71].

Postoperatively, is necessary to apply a plastic brace for six months. In fact, Harrington has shown that several years are required for the spinal fusion to mature and physical activities are restricted for the first two years after operation.

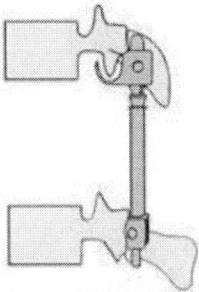

Figure 43. Harrington instrumentation: distraction device is inserted superiorly into the articular facets or lamina and inferiorly into the superior surface of the lamina.

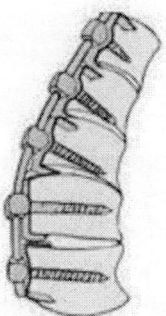

Figure 44. Dwyer instrumentation: staples on the vertebral body with screws inserted through the staples into the vertebra and the cable introduced through the screw heads.

In case of lumbar curves with hyperlordosis or when posterior elements are deficient or congenitally absent, as in myelomeningoceles, is valuable the anterior fusion developed by Dwyer and associates (Figure 44) [72]. Described in 1969, the Dwyer procedure was widely used during the 1970s. The main indication were lumbar idiopathic scoliosis and neurogenic scoliosis, the latter often combined with an additional posterior procedure. The technique consists in a complete excision of the intervertebral discs and addition of bone between the vertebral endplates to achieve an interbody fusion. The instrumentation includes a plate or staple driven to span the vertebral body; a screw inserted through the staple into the vertebra and a cable inserted in the head of the screw.

Dwyer instrumentation must not be performed in the presence of kyphosis, which will be increased by this procedure. Moreover, this operation is not recommended in thorax spine and for patients under the age of 10 years because of the immaturity of the vertebral bodies and the size of the instrumentation. In elderly patients with osteoporosis, the bone is too weak to achieve secure fixation and loss of correction can occur.

For many years, surgical instrumentation for treating scoliosis was designed primarily to apply distraction forces to the spine. The Cotrel-Dubousset instrumentation has provide for application of a complex combination of force to correct the spinal deformity, as well as providing increased rigidity of the final construct. It uses hooks and rods in a cross-linked pattern to realign the spine. Its reported advantages include the ability to obtain three-plane correction of the deformity and to allow immediate postoperative mobilization without an orthosis [73]. It has been reported the risk of creating an iatrogenic flatback deformity with use of posterior instrumentation, which has not demonstrated any consistent ability to normalize sagittal plane deformities.

The reported advantages of Cotrel-Dubousset instrumentation include the ability to obtain three-plane correction of the deformity and allow immediate postoperative mobilization without an orthosis (Figure 45). With Cotrel-Dubousset instrumentation there is the option of applying both selective distraction and compression forces. Also by use of the derotation maneuver there is less reliance on actual distraction than with Harrington instrumentation. Hook placement pattern are determined by force direction required to reconstruct the sagittal plane. Generally, distractive direction forces (away from the apical vertebra) produce kyphosis and compressive direction forces (toward apical vertebra) produce lordosis. Additionally, the concave side can be approached first to produce kyphosis with divergent hooks and convex side first to produce lordosis with convergent direction hooks. The rod on the concave side of the scoliosis is applied first, then it is rotated and locked to the hooks. This "derotation maneuver" is intended to rotate the spine from its predominant plane of curvature in the frontal plane into the sagittal plane, to produce a normal kyphosis or lordosis [74].

So, Cotrel-Dubousset instrumentation has gained acceptance for correction and stabilization of adolescent idiopathic scoliosis because of increased rotational correction. The main advantage of Cotrel-Dubousset instrumentation is that, because of the extensive cross-linking, the patient may not have to wear a cast or brace after surgery. In some cases, the use of Cotrel-Dubousset has been extended to include all scoliosis, even those neurologically involved patients with larger, stiffer curves. The disadvantage is the complexity of the operation and the number of hooks and cross links.

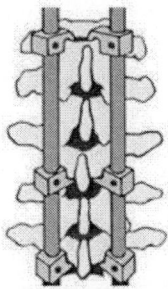

Figure 45. Cotrel-Dubousset instrumentation: hooks and rods in a cross-linked pattern to realign the spine and redistribute the biomechanical stresses.

Conclusion

At present we cannot exclude other factors than the above can influence the estrogen effects on bone metabolism. However, the teenagers affected by IS, show in all cases lower levels of steroids when compared to teenagers that do not show the IS phenotype. We postulate that there is a linkage between IS phenotype and endocrine status of teenagers affect by the disease, and that the IS show a clear cut sex-dependent manifestation. It is clear that a great deal remains to be learned about the idiopathic scoliosis. The mechanism of production of spinal curvature remains unclear. We hope that the genetic aspects of the disease may be clarified so that the disease can be prevented rather than treated by troublesome braces or extensive surgery.

References

[1] F. Adams. Hippocrates: The genuine works of Hippocrates. 1849; London.

[2] F.R. Packard. Life and Times of Ambroise Paré. Ed 2. New York, P. B. Hoeber ed. 1926.

[3] N. Andry. Orthopaedia. London, A. Millar ed. 1743.

[4] R.A. Hibbs. An operation for progressive spinal deformities. A preliminary report of three cases from the service of the New York Orthopaedic Hospital. *New York Med. J.* 1911; 1013.
[5] W.P. Blount. Scoliosis and the Milwaukee brace. *Bull Hosp. Joint Dis.* 1958; 19: 152-165.
[6] W.P. Blount and A.C. Schmidt. The Milwaukee brace in the treatment of scoliosis. *Proc. Am. Acad. Orthop. Surg. J. Bone Joint Surg.* 1957; 39A: 693.
[7] J.H. Moe. Methods and techniques of evaluating idiopathic scoliosis. A.A.O.S., Symposium on the Spine, 1967: 196-240. St Louis, C.V. Mosby ed.
[8] A.F. Dwyer: An anterior approach in scoliosis. A preliminary report. *Clin. Orthop.* 1969; 62: 192.
[9] R.L. Dewald and R.D. Ray. Skeletal traction for the treatment of severe scoliosis. *J. Bone Joint Surg.* 1970; 52A: 233-238.
[10] J.R. Cobb. Outline for the study of scoliosis. *Am. Acad. Orthop. Surgeons Lect.* 1948; 5: 261.
[11] I.V. Ponseti and D. Friedman. Prognosis in idiopathic scoliosis. *J. Bone Joint Surg.* 1950; 32A: 381-395.
[12] C. Nash and J. Moe. A study of vertebral rotation. *J. Bone Joint Surg.,* 1969; 51A: 223.
[13] J.R. Cobb. Outline for study of scoliosis: in Instructional course lectures, the American Academy of Orthopaedic surgeons. 1948; vol. 5 Ann Arbor, Mich., J.W. Edwards Co. ed.
[14] W.W. Greulich and S.I. Pyle. Radiographic Atlas of Skeletal Development of the Hand and Wrist. 1959; 2nd ed. Stanford, Calif., Stanford University Press).
[15] J.S. Risser. The iliac apophysis: An invaluable sign in the management of scoliosis. *Clin. Orthop.* 1958; 11: 111.
[16] P. Stagnara. Les déformations du rachis. 1985; Masson, Paris.
[17] J.I.P. James. Kyphoscoliosis. *J. Bone Jont Surg.* 1955; 37B: 414.
[18] H.L. Brooks, S.P. Azen, E. Gerberg, R. Brooks and L. Chan. Scoliosis: A prospective epidemiological study. *J. Bone Joint Surg.* 1975; 57A: 969-972.
[19] R.J. Rogala, D.S. Drummond and J. Gurr. Scoliosis: incidence and natural story. *J. Bone Joint Surg.* 1978: 60A: 172-176.
[20] P.R. Harrington. The etiology of idiopathic scoliosis. *Clin. Orthop.* 1977; 126: 17-25.

[21] E.J. Riseborough, R. Wynne-Davies. A genetic survey of idiopathic scoliosis in Boston, Massacchussetts. *J. Bone Joint Surg. Am* 1973; 55: 974-82.
[22] C.M. Justice, N.H. Miller, B.M.S. Marosy, J. Zhang, A.F. Wilson. Familial Idiopathic Scoliosis: evidence of an X-linked susceptibility locus. *Spine* 2003; 6:589-594.
[23] A.J. Carr. Adolescent idiopathic scoliosis in identical twins. *J. Bone Joint Surg. Br* 1990; 72: 1077.
[24] K.L. Kesling, K.A. Reinker. Scoliosis in twins: a meta-analysis of the literature and report of six cases. *Spine* 1997; 22: 2009-15.
[25] H.R. Cowell, J.N. Hall, G.D. MacEwen. Genetic aspects of idiopathic scoliosis: a Nicholas Andry Award essay, 1970. *Clin. Orthop.* 1972; 86: 121-31.
[26] N.A. Filho, M.W .Thompson. Genetic studies in scoliosis. *J. Bone Joint Surg. Am* 1971; 53: 199.
[27] N.H. Miller, P.D. Sponseller, J. Bell. Genomic search for X-linkage in familial adolescent idiopathic scoliosis. In: Stokes IAF, ed. Research Into Spinal Deformities, 2nd ed. Amsterdam: IOS Press, 1999: 209-13.
[28] A. Czeizel, A. Bellyei, O. Barta. Genetics of adolescent idiopathic scoliosis. *J. Med. Genet.* 1978; 15: 424-7.
[29] T.I. Axenovich, A.M. Zaidman, I.V. Zorkolseve. Segregation analysis of idiopathic scoliosis: evidence for a major-gene effect. *Am. J. Med. Genet.* 1999; 86: 389-94.
[30] V. Chan, C.Y.G. Fong, K.D. Luk, B. Yip, M.K. Lee, M.S. Wong, D.D.S. Lu, and T.W. Chan. A genetic locus for adolescent idiopathic scoliosis linked to chromosome 19p13.3. *Am. J. Hm. Genet.* 2002; 71:401-6.
[31] C.A. Wise, R. Barnes, J. Gillum. Localization of susceptibility to familial idiopathic scoliosis. *Spine* 2000; 25: 2372-80.
[32] L.B. Salehi, M. Mangino, S. De Serio. Assignment of a locus for autosomal idiopathic scoliosis (IS) to human chromosome 17p11. *Hum. Genet.* 2002; 111:401-4.
[33] N.H. Miller, C.M. Justice, B. Marosy, K.F. Doheny, E. Pugh, J. Zhang, H.C. Dietz, A.F. Wilson. Identification of candidate regions for familial idiopathic scoliosis. *Spine* 2005; 30: 1181–1187.
[34] W.H. Kruskal and W. A. Wallis. Use of ranks in one-criterion variance analysis. *J. Am. Statistical Ass*. 1952; 47: 583–621.
[35] H. Levene. Robust tests for equality of variances. In I. Olkin, H. Hotelling. *Stanford University Press*. 1960 pp. 278–292.

[36] S. Moverare, K. Venken, A.L. Eriksson, N. Andersson, S. Skrtic, J. Wergedal, S.Mohan, P. Salmon, R. Bouillon, J.A. Gustafsson, D. Vanderschueren, C. Ohlsson. Differential effects on bone of estrogen receptor_ and androgen receptor activation in orchidectomized adult male mice. *PNAS* 2003;100 13573–13578.

[37] G.A. Greendale, S. Edelstein, E. Barrett-Connor, Endogenous sex steroids and bone mineral density in older women and men: the Rancho Bernardo study. *J. Bone Miner Res.* 1997; 12: 1833–1843.

[38] C.W. Slemenda, C. Longcope, L. Zhou, S.L. Hui, M. Peacock, C.C. Johnston, Sex steroids and bone mass in older men. Positive associations with serum estrogens and negative associations with androgens. *J. Clin. Invest.* 1997; 100: 1755–1759.

[39] S. Khosla, L.J. Melton 3rd, E.J. Atkinson, W.M. O'Fallon, G.G. Klee, B.L. Riggs, Relationship of serum sex steroid levels and bone turnover markers with bone mineral density in men andwomen: a key role for bioavailable estrogen. *J. Clin. Endocrinol. Metab.* 1998; 83: 2266–2274.

[40] B. Ongphiphadhanakul, R. Rajatanavin, S. Chanprasertyothin, N. Piaseu, L. Chailurkit, Serum oestradiol and oestrogen-receptor gene polymorphism are associated with bone mineral density independently of serum testosterone in normal males. *Clin. Endocrinol.* 1998; 49: 803–809.

[41] J.R. Center, T.V. Nguyen, P.N. Sambrook, J.A. Eisman, Hormonal and biochemical parameters in the determination of osteoporosis in elderly men. *J. Clin. Endocrinol. Metab.* 1999; 84: 3626–3635.

[42] S. Amin, Y. Zhang, C.T. Sawin, S.R. Evans, M.T. Hannan, D.P. Kiel, P.W. Wilson, D.T. Felson. Association of hypogonadism and estradiol levels with bone mineral density in elderly men from the Framingham study. *Ann. Int. Med.* 2000; 133: 951–963.

[43] A.W. van den Beld, F.H. de Jong, D.E. Grobbee, H.A. Pols, S.W. Lamberts, Measures of bioavailable serum testosterone and estradiol and their relationships with muscle strength, bone density, and body composition in elderly men. *J. Clin. Endocrinol. Metab.* 2000; 85: 3276–3282.

[44] P. Szulc, F. Munoz, B. Claustrat, P. Garnero, F. Marchand, F. Duboeuf, P.D. Delmas, Bioavailable estradiolmay be animportant determinant of osteoporosis in men: the MINOS study. *J. Clin. Endocrinol. Metab.* 2001; 86 192–199.

[45] D. Mellstrom, O. Johnell, O. Ljunggren, A.L. Eriksson, M. Lorentzon, H. Mallmin, A. Holmberg, I. Redlund-Johnell, E. Orwoll, C. Ohlsson.

Free testosterone is an independent predictor of BMD and prevalent fractures in elderly men: MrOS Sweden, *J. Bone Miner Res.* 2006; 21: 529–535.
[46] A.B. Araujo, T.G. Travison, B.Z. Leder, J.B. McKinlay, Correlations between serum testosterone, estradiol, and sex hormone-binding globulin and bone mineral density in a diverse sample of men. *J. Clin. Endocrinol. Metab.* 2008; 93: 2135–2141.
[47] S. Khosla, L.J. Melton 3rd, E.J. Atkinson,W.M. O'Fallon, Relationship of serum sex steroid levels to longitudinal changes in bone density in young versus elderly men. *J. Clin. Endocrinol. Metab.* 2001; 86: 3555–3561.
[48] C. Carani, K. Qin, M. Simoni, M. Faustini-Fustini, S. Serpente, J. Boyd, K.S. Korach, E.R. Simpson, Effect of testosterone and estradiol in a man with aromatase deficiency. *N. Engl. J. Med.* 1997; 337: 91–95.
[49] J.P. Bilezikian, A. Morishima, J. Bell, M.M. Grumbach, Increased bone mass as a result of estrogen therapy in a man with aromatase deficiency. *N. Engl. J. Med.* 1998; 339: 599–603.
[50] F. Lanfranco, L. Zirilli, M. Baldi, E. Pignatti, G. Corneli, E. Ghigo, G. Aimaretti, C. Carani, V. Rochira, A novel mutation in the human aromatase gene: insights on the relationship among serum estradiol, longitudinal growth and bone mineral density in an adult man under estrogen replacement treatment. *Bone* 2008; 43: 628–635.
[51] V. Rochira, M. Faustini-Fustini, A. Balestrieri, C. Carani, Estrogen replacement therapy in a man with congenital aromatase deficiency: effects of different doses of transdermal estradiol on bone mineral density and hormonal parameters. *J. Clin. Endocrinol. Metab.* 2000; 85: 1841–1845.
[52] T.Esposito, R. Uccello, R. Caliendo, G.F. Di Martino, U.A. Gironi Carnevale, S. Cuomo, D. Ronca, B. Varriale. Estrogen receptor polymorphism, estrogen content and idiopathic scoliosis in human: A possible genetic linkage. *J Steroid Biochem Mol Biol* 2009; 116: 56-60.
[53] K. Venken, K. De Gendt, S. Boonen, J. Ophoff, R. Bouillon, J.V. Swinnen, G. Verhoeven, D. Vanderschueren, Relative impact of androgen and estrogen receptor activation in the effects of androgens on trabecular and cortical bone in growing male mice: a study in the androgen receptor knockout mouse model, *J. Bone Miner Res.* 2006; 21: 576–585.
[54] M.K. Lindberg, S.Moverare, S. Skrtic, S. Alatalo, J. Halleen, S. Mohan, J.A. Gustafsson, C. Ohlsson, Two different pathways for the

maintenance of trabecular bone in adult male mice. *J. Bone Miner Res.* 2002; 17: 555–562.
[55] M.K. Lindberg, S.L. Alatalo, J.M. Halleen, S. Mohan, J.A. Gustafsson, C. Ohlsson, Estrogen receptor specificity in the regulation of the skeleton in female mice. *J. Endocrinol.* 2001; 171: 229–236.
[56] M.K. Lindberg, Z. Weihua, N. Andersson, S. Moverare, H. Gao, O. Vidal, M. Erlandsson, S. Windahl, G. Andersson, D.B. Lubahn, H. Carlsten, K. Dahlman-Wright, J.A. Gustafsson, C. Ohlsson, Estrogen receptor specificity for the effects of estrogen in ovariectomized mice. *J. Endocrinol.* 2002; 174: 167–178.
[57] N.A. Sims, P. Clement-Lacroix, D. Minet, C. Fraslon-Vanhulle, M. Gaillard-Kelly, M. Resche-Rigon, R. Baron, A functional androgen receptor is not sufficient to allow estradiol to protect bone after gonadectomy in estradiol receptordeficient mice. *J. Clin. Invest.* 2003; 111: 1319–1327.
[58] N.A. Sims, S. Dupont, A. Krust, P. Clement-Lacroix, D. Minet, M. Resche-Rigon, M. Gaillard-Kelly, R. Baron, Deletion of estrogen receptors reveals a regulatory role for estrogen receptors-beta in bone remodelling in females but not in males. *Bone* 2002; 30: 18–25.
[59] M.H. Harynk, S.A.W. Fuqua, Estroger receptor mutations in human desease. *Endocrinol. Rev.* 2004; 25: 869–898.
[60] A. Nachemson. A long-term follow-up study of non treated scoliosis. *Acta Orthop. Scand.* 1968; 39: 466.
[61] G.E. Thomas. Idiopathic scoliosis. *J. Bone Joint Surg.* 1947; 29: 907.
[62] J.H. Moe, R.B. Winter, D.S. Bradford, J.E. Lonstein. Scoliosis and other deformity. 1978; W.B. Saunders Company.
[63] J.E. Lonstein, J.M. Carlson. The prediction of curve progression in untreated idiopathic scoliosis during growth. *J. Bone Joint Surg.* 1984; 66A: 1061-1071.
[64] W.P. Blount, A.C. Schmidt, E.D. Keever, E.T. Leonard. The Milwaukee brace in the operative treatment of scoliosis. *J. Bone Joint Surg.* 1968; 40A: 511.
[65] J.H. Moe, D.N. Kettleson. Idiopathic scoliosis analysis of curve patterns and preliminary results of Milwaukee brace treatment in 169 patients. *J. Bone Joint Surg.* 1970; 52A: 1500.
[66] A. Nordwall. Strides in idiopathic scoliosis. *Acta Orthop Scand* 1973; Suppl. 150.
[67] J. Cotrel J. and G. Morel. La technique de l'E.D.F. dans las corretction des scoliosis. *Rev. Chr. Orthop.* 1964; 50: 59.

[68] C.R. Michel, G. Allègre, P. Schuster, M. Onimus. Traitement des scoliosis lombaires évolutives. *Rev. Chir. Orthop.* 1977; 63 (Suppl II): 31-37.

[69] J.E. Hall, W. Miller, W. Shuman, W. Stanish. A refined concept in the orthotic management of idiopathic scoliosis. *Prosthet. Orthot. Int.* 1975; 29: 7-13.

[70] J.B. Emans, A. Kaelin, P.H. Bancel, J.E. Hall and M.E. Miller. The Boston bracing system for idiopathic scoliosis. Follow-up results in 295 patients. *Spine* 1986; 11: 792-801.

[71] P.R. Harrington. Treatment of scoliosis. Correction and internal fixation by spine instrumentation. *J. Bone Joint Surg.* 1962; 44A: 591.

[72] A.F. Dwyer. Experience of anterior correction of scoliosis. Clin. Orthop. 1973; 93: 191.

[73] J.P. Thompson, E.E. Transfeldt, D.S. Bradford, J.W. Ogilvie, O. Boachie-Adjei. Decompensation after Cotre-Dubousset instrumentation of idiopathic scoliosis. *Spine* 1990; 15: 927-941.

[74] K.H. Bridwell, B. Randall, A.M. Capelli, G. Huss, C. Harvey. Sagittal plane analysis in idiopathic scoliosis patients treated with Cotrel-Dubousset instrumentation. *Spine* 1990; 15: 921-926.

In: Scoliosis: Causes, Symptoms and Treatment ISBN: 978-1-62081-007-1
Editors: A. Bessette et al. © 2012 Nova Science Publishers, Inc.

Chapter II

Scoliosis, Orthodontics and Occlusion, Are There Evidence?

Amat Philippe
Department of Orthodontics, Paris, France
Member of the editorial boards of the
Revue d'Orthopedie Dento-Faciale and L'Orthodontie Française.
Associate Editor of the L'Orthodontie Française, France

Abstract

This presentation addresses the questions raised by the connections between idiopathic scoliosis, orthodontics and occlusion, as well as their therapeutic implications.

Idiopathic scoliosis makes its appearance before the end of the growth period, unassociated with other pathologies, which also differentiates them from scoliosis that are secondary to other problems such as malformations and neurological disorders. The etiology of idiopathic scoliosis is probably multifactorial, with components that are hormonal, connected with growth, with genetics, with metabolic disturbances of collagens and proteoglycanes, with neurological disturbances, and with biomechanical factors.

How should orthodontists deal with patients who suffer from idiopathic scoliosis? Does the malady exert a pernicious effect on the patient's occlusion? Will orthodontic treatment ameliorate or aggravate the patient's over-all health? These are the principal questions that must be answered when patients with scoliosis seek an orthodontic consultation.

To answer these questions, we conducted a comprehensive review of the literature, which shows that there is a lack of reliable publications devoted to this subject. Most publications devoted to the relations between scoliosis, orthodontics and occlusion have been prepared with meager methodological rigor which makes it difficult to derive a clear answer from them to the questions that we have just outlined.

The data that is available points to the existence of a correlation between posture and occlusion and also asserts the prevalence of associations between cranio-facial anomalies and idiopathic scoliosis in adolescents.

The strong prevalence of associations between scoliosis and cranio-facial anomalies argues persuasively for the related disciplines of general orthopedics and dento-facial orthopedics to work cooperatively in early diagnosis of patients an in increasing the effectiveness of the treatment of those patients.In this way orthodontists could contribute to the orthopedist ' s beginning early treatment of spinal cord deformities by suggesting an orthopedic consultation when orthodontic examinations have uncovered certain indicative dento-skeletal characteristics such as Class II malocclusion or dento-facial asymmetry.Cases of idiopathic scoliosis often develop in unpredictable ways during growth periods. Not infrequently, the malady may become more grave or, in other cases, stabilize during the time a patient is undergoing orthodontic treatment and the orthodontist' s mechano-therapy may be blamed or given credit. This, of course would affirm without a shred of proof that an association between two phenomena establishes a cause and effect relationship between them.To find more answers we need to undertake basic and clinical research projects that could eventually establish the validity of a cause and effect relationship between dental occlusion and posture that would put therapy on evidence-based foundation.

1. Introduction

It is probably fair to say that the inter-relationship between occlusion, orthodontics and scoliosis (and more generally posture), are of interest for a significant number of practitioners. However, a certain amount of confusion surrounds this connection because of the wide diversity of therapeutic approaches designed to deal with it and the weakness of methodological design in the scientific studies that have been published on it to date.

The inter-actions between scoliosis, orthodontics and occlusion constitute a vast topic. With this presentation we hope to stimulate discussion and thinking about it and suggest that scientific study can often corroborate our original unsubstantiated convictions.

The inter-actions between idiopathic scoliosis, orthodontics and occlusion are parts of the larger issue of the inter-relationship between orthodontics, occlusion and posture.

2. Occlusion and Posture: A Reciprocal Inter-Change

2.1. Definitions

Our subject is dental occlusion. The dictionary of orthognathics[21] published by the Société Française d'Orthopédie Dento-Faciale defines it as a phrase in current use employed to described the reciprocal action of the dental arches

The same tome offers a double definition of posture:

- The habitual stance of the body or parts of it supported by the action and constraints of tonic muscles that work to fix the body segments through joints designed to maintain equilibrium.
- Bodily stance derived from the interaction of bodily weight and the sensori-motor complex (derived from the labyrinth of the inner ear, the Pacini bodies, the Golgi apparatus, the joints, the plantar surfaces of the feet.

2.2. Posture and Dento-Facial Orthopedics

Orthodontists should take a consistent and on-going interest in the posture of their patients. In addition to the establishment of the dental objectives of their mechano-therapy they should also be attentive to the eventual relationship between occlusion and cephalic as well as over-all bodily posture, taking into account physiological regulation of varying mandibulo-cranial positions. It is equally important that they consider the interaction between cranio-cervical posture and cranio-facial morphogenesis[80].

Clinically, orthodontists have to face with a number of questions. In the first place, they find that interest bearing on the relationship between occlusion and posture leads them into a battleground with at least two fronts. Patients consult them seeking occlusal treatment that they hope, or have been told by practitioners in allied fields, will help to improve their postural problems. How should we respond to these requests? Our patients have a right not to be deprived of effective treatment, no matter what it might be. They also have the right to benefit from true informed consent and we have the obligation to tell them exactly what medical benefit they can expect to derive from therapy, especially if that therapy is invasive. In other words, they have a right to be presented with a clear cost/benefit/risk analysis.

3. Occlusion and Posture: Facts and Beliefs

3.1. The Indispensable Evidence-Based Approach

Designed to help us achieve a global improvement in the quality of our treatment and to bridge the gap between clinical research and the health care we deliver, the evidence-based approach[70, 71] has been widely accepted in the medical community.

Evidence-based dento-facial orthopedics[7, 8] describes the application of factual data to our specialty. Let us emphasize that its three components, clinical experience, the best available published data on clinical research, and the values and preferences of our patients, must be welded together so that orthodontists and their patients can cooperate fully in a *diagnostic and therapeutic alliance*. The most thorough going review of the literature devoted to the postural approach will, unfortunately, deal with a limited number of controlled studies carried out with methodological rigor.

3.2. Occlusion and Posture: What Does Appear in the Literature?

3.2.1. The Questions

In addition to the simple issue of the existence of a relationship between occlusion and posture, several other questions have been posed.

What are the criteria for normal posture of the body, the head and the spinal column, and the mandibulo-cranial complex? Are these criteria valid?

How should malfunctions of posture be defined? What are the consequences of the malfunctions structurally, in causing pain, and can they be evaluated in terms of deficiency, of incapacity, or of handicap[4]? And have the results of postural treatment been confirmed by controlled studies?

Clinicians should also ask themselves about the nature of the mechanisms of the regulation of posture and the limits of postural adaptation. Is orthodontic treatment a contributing factor to the etiology of postural deformities or isn't it? Can changes in occlusion affect, in a clinically significant manner, global postural equilibrium? Can occlusion actually provoke postural disturbances or pathological ailments in sites far distant from the oral cavity?

Variations in dental occlusion are manifold and appear in a variety of ways; malformations, attrition due to function or faulty habits, irregularities of teeth, and changes resulting from dental restorations, orthodontic care, and prosthetic rehabilitation. What eventual influence does each of these have on postural balance?

Finally, another interrogation is based on the possible role that dento-facial orthopedic therapy could have in the treatment of postural disorders.

3.2.2. The Weakness of Published Data

Most publications devoted to the relations between posture and occlusion have been prepared with meager methodological rigor which makes it difficult to derive a clear answer from them to the questions that we have just outlined.

To answer these questions, a comprehensive review of the literature. The literature survey was performed by applying the Medline database (Entrez PubMed, www.ncbi.nim.nih.gov). The survey covered the period from January 1966 to to october 2011. The headings sequence "Posture" [MeSH] AND " Dental occlusion "[MeSH] was selected. Additionally, a search in the Cochrane Clinical Trials Register (www.cochrane.org/reviews) was performed. The titles and abstracts of all potentially relevant articles were reviewed. Electronic searches were followed up with secondary searches.

The search strategy resulted in 371 articles. 24 of them were reviews. Seven RCTs were retrieved.

In any assessment it is quite clear that a great many of the articles dealing with the relationship between occlusion and posture are anecdotal reports of clinical cases that have little status as scientific evidence.

The scientific studies that have been devoted to the relationship of occlusion to posture suffer, as a group, from a variety of flaws[37]. We can site the non-random separation of patients into groups to be studied, the failure, at the close of the study, to measure all of the patients that had participated in the trial, or, to put it in another way, the omission of some of the participants. We should add the frequent defect of poor definition of the criteria for inclusion or exclusion of subjects, the use of patient samples too small in size, and the failure to carefully define the validity of the tests employed with regard to their sensitivity, specificity, and reproducibility.

To find more answers we need to undertake basic and clinical research projects that could eventually establish the validity of a cause and effect relationship between dental occlusion and posture that would put therapy on evidence based foundation[23,24].

3.2.3. A Few Comments

The difficulties that participants in this field have had in obtaining experimental results that are clearly reliable should not prevent us from discerning in this bewildering jumble the existence of many suggestive implications. Some of the indications we might draw from them are:

- changes in the position of the mandible influence body posture[73];
- reciprocally, body posture seems to have an affect on the position of the mandible[73], with the exception of centric relation and occlusion with maximum inter-cuspation, the localization and reproducibility of both of which are not affected[20, 84];
- habitual mandibular position, or rest position, is tied to cephalic posture[89];
- head posture seems to influence occlusion[74, 75]. It does influence the trajectory of closing, and the position of the initial occlusal contacts[17, 22, 54, 80]. On the other hand, a forward inclined head posture does not appear to have any effect on initial occlusal contacts[52];
- can occlusion affect the way feet support weight? The conclusions of published studies on the point are contradictory. Ferrario et al.[29] have shown that adjustments of the centers of pressure in the feet are not influenced by pain felt in the masticatory system, Class II subdivision malocclusions, or by variations in occlusal positioning. But other studies[14, 15] do assert that the occlusion exerts an influence on the pressures applied through the feet;
- many studies refer to a supposed correlation between malfunction of the masticatory apparatus and an anterior positioning of the head[16, 47, 48, 81]. These correlations should make clinicians consider the

- advisability of integrating the evaluation and treatment of postural defects at the same time they are correcting discrepancies in the masticatory system[16, 43, 45];
- but the results reported in another article[60] do not confirm the hypothesis that body posture provokes or aggravates masticatory discrepancies. Still this work should be evaluated with extreme caution because of the small size of the sample and the large number of postural variables it dealt with;
- the studies that Perinetti carried out using a stabilometric platform did not produce any evidence that there was a correlation between dental occlusion and bodily posture[63], nor that patients with TMJ problems had perforce alterations in bodily posture[64];
- patients suffering from internal derangement of the temporo-mandibular joint do not necessarily hold their heads in an advanced position[39];
- pain felt in the masticatory apparatus is not associated with cephalic posture[86];
- a recent systematic review of the literature suggests that the hypothesis that there is a relationship between cervico-cephalic posture and disorders of the masticatory process remains uncertain[10];
- many articles claim to show that there is a relationship between cervico-cephalic posture and cranio-facial morphology. Cervical posture appears to be strongly correlated with structural variations in the sagittal and vertical dimensions of the face11, [26]. Positive correlations have also been demonstrated between cervico-cephalic posture and both mandibular and maxillary anterior dento-alveolar height as well as with the inclinations of the upper and lower occlusal planes[78];
- children with Class III skeletal malocclusions present a significantly lower extent of cervical lordosis than those with skeletal Class I or II occlusions[26];
- on the other hand, children with Class II skeletal malocclusions have significantly increased cervical lordosis compared with children with Class I or II occlusions[26], and subjects in Class II keep their heads more forward to a significant extent[34];

- a study conducted using a posturographic platform showed that subjects in Class II had body posture projected forward and those with Class III malocclusions a bodily posture projected backward[61];
- a negative correlation exists between cervical lordosis and mandibular length[31];
- many studies seem to indicate that the afferent impulses of the trigeminal participate in the relationship of occlusion and postural regulation[35, 36]. They allege that there is an inter-dependence between the sensory and motor innervations of the trigeminal nerve and the cervical complex[18];
- there is a significant association between the dominant eye and homolateral rotation of the head. In patients suffering from discrepancies of the masticatory system there is also a significant association between the side of the cephalic rotation and a contra-lateral deviation of the mandibular incisive midline[66];
- In a study conducted by P. Gangloff of participants in riflery sports[35], the stabilization of sight was found to have an effect on postural control through mediation of the dental occlusion ;
- Michelotti et al[56] studied patients with posterior cross bites using a stabilometer platform and found in two modalities, occlusion at maximum inter-cuspation and a position with teeth held comfortably apart with cotton rolls. They found the cross bites had no effect on the stability of bodily posture. They concluded that there would be no justification for correcting the cross bites if the objective were to prevent or treat a postural problem.
- in addition, another study found that posterior cross bites were not correlated with inequality in leg length of young adolescents[57];
- an excessive cranio-cervical angulation is associated with lower anterior crowding[3, 79]. This conclusion is in accord with a hypothesis about stretching of soft tissues according to which patients with extended cranio-cervical posture have a blockage of the sagittal growth of their dental arches from the dorsal tension exerted on them;
- does muscular force vary with the occlusion? Maximal biting force is greater when the head is extended than it is when the head is held in a natural position[41].
- a splint that places the mandible in a position determined by kinesiological tests would be likely to augment muscular force1, [32, 33]. These results contradict those of another published article that

avers that there is no correlation between biting force and cephalic posture[82].
- Kovero et al. also did not find any significant statistical correlation between maximal biting force and cervical posture[46];
- the neuromuscular activity of neck and face muscles seems to influence corporal or bodily posture according to many studies[25, 58, 59, 76], but, according to another one, do not[85];
- bruxism could be associated with a head posture that is inclined excessively downward and forward[87];
- a recent systematic review of the literature[40] surveys 266 publications reporting on a relationship between the masticatory apparatus and disturbances of the spinal column. There is an interrelation between the masticatory apparatus and head posture according to 216 articles, and an association between pelvic tilting and the oral cavity according to 53 studies. 131 articles conclude that the occlusion affects posture and 171 assert that posture affects occlusion.

These reports from the extensive literature suggest that our mechanotherapies can have an effect on the bodily posture of our patients. But because of the widespread lack of methodological rigor in these investigations, orthodontists should examine the results with prudence and circumspection, especially in view of their tendency to be mutually contradictory. By doing this we can avoid the risk of over-treating our patients by being scrupulously critical when we add postural considerations to our diagnoses[40].

4. The Special Case of the Relationship between Idiopathic Scoliosis and Occlusion in Adolescents

When a diagnosis of idiopathic scoliosis is made, patients are confronted with the possibility that their spines will continue to develop in a deformed way until the end of the growth period. The best outcome for them would be merely to have to submit to regular check-up examinations about the state of the vertebral column. But some of them will have to endure especially grave orthopedic or surgical treatment. Because of the seriousness of the global effect of the disorder and its esthetic, psychological, and functional repercussions a close study of idiopathic scoliosis helps to answer many questions that arise about the interrelations between posture and occlusion.

4.1. Idiopathic Scoliosis and Adolescents

Scoliosis is a three-dimensional structural deformation of the spinal column, with rotation of some vertebrae that causes gibbosities. These deformations cannot be totally corrected, which differentiates them from simple tendencies toward scoliosis. Idiopathic scoliosis makes its appearance before the end of the growth period, unassociated with other pathologies, which also differentiates them from scolioses that are secondary to other problems such as malformations and neurological disorders.

Conventionally, idiopathic scoliosis is called infantile if it is detected before the child is three years old and juvenile if it appears clinically in children from three to ten.

When scoliosis appears in children between the age of ten and the time of skeletal maturation it is said to be adolescent, a category that embraces 80% of the ensemble of cases of idiopathic scoliosis[88]. Affecting more girls than boys, the disorder[67] is seen in about 2 to 4% of adolescents between the ages of 10 to 16.

The etiology of idiopathic scoliosis is probably multi-factorial, with components that are hormonal, connected with growth, with genetics, with metabolic disturbances of collagens and proteoglycanes, with neurological disturbances especially of the proprioceptive and equilibration systems, and with biomechanical factors[19, 68].

With regular clinical and radiological examinations the progress of the malady can be observed. According to Lonstein and Carlson[51], the topography of the individual case of scoliosis, the patient's age at the time it was discerned, the initial degree of angulation, the results of the Risser test, and, for girls, the date of the onset of menstruation, can all be evaluated as factors in the "prediction of curvature progression in untreated idiopathic scoliosis during growth." Treatment of evolving idiopathic scoliosis is usually conservative at first having the objective improving the appearance and the functioning of the spinal column and preventing any aggravation of the curvatures that have already occurred. Some patients are asked to wear braces that are adjusted to various degrees of correction. When the malady progresses unfavorably and the deformation becomes more serious, surgical treatment may be indicated. But, throughout, careful observation of the patients and their families is of primordial importance because the necessary procedures can be long, tedious, and extremely constraining. The primary goal with all patients is to limit the development of the scoliosis so that it does not become a serious impediment to a normal, active life when patients become adults.

4.2. Adolescents with Idiopathic Scoliosis and Orthodontic Treatment

How should orthodontists deal with patients who suffer from idiopathic scoliosis? Does the malady exert a pernicious effect on the patient's occlusion? Will orthodontic treatment ameliorate or aggravate the patient's over-all health? These are the principal questions that must be answered when patients with scoliosis seek an orthodontic consultation.

Cases of idiopathic scoliosis often develop in unpredictable ways during growth periods. Not infrequently, the malady may become more grave or, in other cases, stabilize[38] during the time a patient is undergoing orthodontic treatment and the orthodontist's mechano-therapy may be blamed or given credit. This, of course would affirm without a shred of proof that an association between two phenomena establishes a cause and effect relationship between them.

This calls to mind a parallel between another debate that caused a considerable stir in orthodontic circles during the 1980s when orthodontic treatment was alleged to have caused some patients tempero-mandibular disorders or so-called TMJ problems. During the epidemic of this unfortunate witch hunt some patients actually obtained substantial financial awards[65] for alleged malpractice. Fortunately a series of subsequent clinical studies[55] was able to prove that dento-facial orthopedic treatment did not increase the risk of a patient's developing tempero-mandibular maladies.

We have derived the answer to the series of questions we posed by means of a virtual dialogue between members of diverse health disciplines in an attempt to restore some unity to the evaluation of patients whose examinations are too often fragmented into studies of separate organs to fit the vision of a host of medical specialties and by a careful study of the literature.

4.3. The Occlusion of Adolescents with Idiopathic Scoliosis: What Does the Published Data Tell Us?

Many studies have been carried out to try to determine if a scoliotic deformation can be associated not only with adaptive asymmetries of postural control but also with a particular type dento-skeletal formation.

4.3.1. Does Treatment of Scoliosis Tend to Affect a Patient's Dento-Facial Equilibrium?

During the decades of the 1960 and 70s many articles were published about the deleterious effects on facial growth that orthopedic treatment of scoliosis with a Milwaukee brace could cause.

In a 1966 article R. G. Alexander[2] presented evidence that there was a significant reduction of facial height, an elevation of the palatal plane, a flattening of the palatal vault, a tilting, lower and forward, of the mandibular symphasis, intruding of molars, and labial tilting of maxillary and mandibular incisors during treatment of scoliosis with the Milwaukee brace.

Other authorities subsequently suggested that patients wear a variety of appliances, such as the monobloc, to counteract the adverse oro-facial effects of the Milwaukee brace[69].

Because of these studies the Milwaukee brace was then modified so that it would be less likely to provoke unwelcome iatrogenic side effects[49, 53]. More recently Huggare et al[42] described the less substantial side effects of orthopedic treatment for scoliotic patients undertaken with a Boston brace. These patients were distinguished from a control group by an accentuation of the cranio-cervical angle, a rotation of the orbital plane, maxillary, and mandibular planes, a displacement of the mid-line of the mandibular arch, and a flattening of the posterior arch of the first cervical vertebra associated with a lengthening of the *dent de l'axis*.

4.3.2. Correlation between Idiopathic Scoliosis and Dento-Skeletal Characteristics

Pećina M et al. have classified orthodontic anomalies into two categories, hereditary and acquired. They show that in scoliotic patients[62] there is a higher rate of occurrence of *hereditary orthodontic* anomalies like hypodontia, which is 10 times more frequent and prognathic mandibles. On the other hand, these authors did not find a higher incidence of *acquired orthodontic* anomalies in scoliosis patients. They suggest that early detection of hereditary orthodontic discrepancies would allow health care givers to identify a group of infants with a high risk of later developing scoliosis.

Lippold et al. found a statistically significant correlation between Class II malocclusion and scoliosis[50].

They recommend that all pre-school children with Class II malocclusions, no matter how slight, should be carefully watched for possible development of spinal abnormalities.

The authors of another article[44] conclude that there is a correlation between skeletal anomalies of Class I, II, or III, hypo or hyper-divergent, and scoliosis.

The study that Ben-Bassat et al[12] published showed patients with scoliosis had more than an average amount of asymmetries in the sagittal and transverse dimensions. Other investigators have observed that patients with scoliosis have prevalence statistically greater than average of Class II subdivision malocclusions, lower incisal mid-line deviations, and, especially, mandibular deviations, as well as anterior and posterior cross bites. On the other hand, no significant correlation has been established between the side to which the spine is deformed and the side of the posterior cross bite or the side to which the mandibular midline is deviated. Some authors do draw our attention to the possibility that the asymmetries of scoliosis and of malocclusion share a common etiology. Should this be true the global correction of a malocclusion, and its retention, could be more uncertain. They advise practitioners examining patients to look for under-lying orthopedic problems when they have made a diagnosis[13] of early signs of dento-facial asymmetry.

Still other workers have studied the relationship between dental occlusion and posture in animals. Festa et al[30] studied the effects in rats of uni-laterally opening their bites by adding composite to posterior teeth. After one week a radiological examination showed a marked deviation of the animals' vertebral columns. When researchers opened the bite similarly on the other side the spinal column straightened up. More recently D'Attilio et al[27] also induced scoliotic curvature in the spinal columns of rats in a week's time by uni-laterally raising the occlusion. When the researchers restored occlusal harmony by elevating the contra-lateral side of the occlusion, vertebral alignment of 83% of the rats in the study returned to the original condition. This seems to make clear that spinal column alignment in rats can be influenced by dental occlusion.

So clinicians are faced with the question of determining to what extent experimental observations made in animal studies can be applied to daily practice. Even if the results of animal studies should not be extrapolated to apply to people but tested on humans first before they are accepted, their conclusions should, at the very least induce practitioners to conduct any mechanical adjustment that could lead to occlusal imbalance with extreme care.

In a recent review, Saccucci et al.[72] evaluated the type of occlusions more prevalent in subjects with scoliosis. They conclude that there is plausible evidence for an increased prevalence of unilateral Angle Class II malocclusions associated with scoliosis, and an increased risk of lateral crossbite, midline deviation in children affected by scoliosis. Also, documentation of associations between reduced range of lateral movements and scoliosis seem convincing.

4.4. Clinical Implications

The strong prevalence of associations between scoliosis and cranio-facial anomalies argues persuasively for the related disciplines of general orthopedics and dento-facial orthopedics to work cooperatively in early diagnosis of patients and in increasing the effectiveness of the treatment of those patients[9].

In this way orthodontists could contribute to the orthopedist's beginning early treatment of spinal cord deformities by suggesting an orthopedic consultation when orthodontic examinations have uncovered certain indicative dento-skeletal characteristics such as Class II malocclusion or dento-facial asymmetry.

It should be emphasized that when orthodontists do not include every facet of their patients' health status in their examinations they may risk missing important diagnostic elements. When they are confronted with a polymorphous symptomology, they must endeavor to assess all of its dimensions including postural in order to avoid parceling treatment into isolated and ineffective components.

Certainly the achievement of a harmonious and esthetic smile for our patients remains one of the objectives of our treatment but the therapeutic perspectives of our specialty go far beyond that. In addition to placing our patients' faces, jaws, and dental arches in better esthetic and functional equilibrium we strive, especially, to re-establish optimal nasal breathing[83], and also to place the soft tissues of the face and the cranio-cervical complex in the best possible postural position.

We need to realize that our patients can be considered entities made of tightly connected psychic and somatic components whose complexity provoked Rudolph Slavicek[77] to propose a cybernetic concept of the mechanism of inter-reaction of the components of the masticatory system. Instead of calling it an apparatus, which designates an ensemble of organs working together in the same function, he prefers the term organism because the masticatory organism fulfills numerous functions. In fact, this ensemble of organs working in a coordinated and hierarchal manner does more than just execute the activities of mastication and deglutition. It also participates in speech, breathing, maintenance of posture, esthetic appearance, and control of emotions and stress. The Central Nervous System regulates these functions not only by neurological somatic control but also by conscious and unconscious psychic interference. R. Slavicek makes a special point of stressing that the methods modern humans use to deal with the pressures and assaults they suffer in daily life often focus on the masticatory organism as an exhaust valve to relieve unconscious psychic charges or stress.

But it is not only desirable but essential that we integrate a postural approach into the practice of dento-facial orthopedics by also including it as a component of *education of patients*.

This attitude of making patient participants in treatment not simple recipients of it, sometimes thought of as *patient education* but, in reality, of far wider scope than that, raises patients to the status of equal partners in the therapeutic enterprise[9]. This demarche can be broken down into three clinical entities that have routinely been described as[28]:

- information about the patient's health;
- information about the patient's malady;
- education about the patient's therapy.

As specialists in caring for the health of children it is highly desirable that orthodontists disseminate all three of these types of information.

Because of the limited amount of space available for this chapter, we haven't been able to discuss the therapeutic education of children in detail. But by at least formulating its three main aspects we wish to emphasize quite explicitly that education of patients is integral part of our treatment. We also strongly believe that instructing them about how to *participate in their therapy,* notably in myo-functional training, especially of breathing, is only one part of the pedagogical relationship between orthodontists and patients that should be a part of every visit. Centered on the patient, these sessions should be adapted to their age and the psycho-social context in which they live and should encompass all the educational aspects of preventive and curative treatment. The goal of this enterprise is to help patients, with the assistance of their families, to acquire the full competence for attaining, among other goals, the capacity for good nasal breathing.

Conclusion

In presenting the correlation between idiopathic scoliosis, orthodontics and dental occlusion published data tends to lend comfortable support for the convictions and clinical impressions we have already formed. The physiological continuum tying occlusion to posture does not appear to be a univocal and linear relationship but instead a complex ensemble made up of numerous contributing factors.

This review of the literature shows that there is a lack of reliable publications devoted to this subject. Most publications devoted to the relations between scoliosis, orthodontics and occlusion have been prepared with meager methodological rigor which makes it difficult to derive a clear answer from them to the questions that we have just outlined.

The data that is available points to the existence of a correlation between posture and occlusion and also asserts the prevalence of associations between cranio-facial anomalies and idiopathic scoliosis in adolescents. This prevalence of associations between scoliosis and cranio-facial anomalies argues persuasively for the related disciplines of general orthopedics and dento-facial orthopedics to work cooperatively in early diagnosis of patients an in increasing the effectiveness of the treatment of those patients.

In this way orthodontists could contribute to the orthopedist ' s beginning early treatment of spinal cord deformities by suggesting an orthopedic consultation when orthodontic examinations have uncovered certain indicative dento-skeletal characteristics such as Class II malocclusion or dento-facial asymmetry.

We must ask ourselves, then, is the frequent association between posture and facial deformities the result of pure coincidence or is it evidence of a real pathological development whose meaning is just beginning to be clarified? With what therapeutic techniques should we deal with these problems? Posing these questions and attempting to answer them is the indispensable pre-requisite for orthodontists to incorporate an evaluation of problems with posture and a consideration of their eventual repercussions in our dento-facial orthopedic treatment. And to find answers we need to undertake basic and clinical research projects that could eventually establish the validity of a cause and effect relationship between dental occlusion and posture without which there can be no sure indications for the directions orthodontic therapy for postural defects should take.

In the final analysis, by including postural considerations in our diagnoses, we shall be moving along the road that leads to a total corporal analysis of our patients. This approach will reinforce our communications with other health care deliverers and encourage us to treat our patients in a multi-disciplinary collaboration with our colleagues in other specialties. We are convinced that such a joint enterprise will be a key element in our common *raison d'etre*: caring for the over-all health and well-being of our patients.

References

[1] Abdallah EF, Mehta NR, Forgione AG, Clark RE. Affecting upper extremity strength by changing maxillo-mandibular vertical dimension in deep bite subjects. *Cranio*, 2004;22:268-75.

[2] Alexander RG. The effects on tooth position and maxillofacial vertical growth during treatment of scoliosis with the Milwaukee brace. *Am. J. Orthod.*, 1966;52:161-89.

[3] AlKofide EA, AlNamankani E. The association between posture of the head and malocclusion in Saudi subjects. *Cranio*, 2007;25:98-105.

[4] Amat P et al. 2001. Evaluation with World Health Organization criterias of TMD and myofascial disorders. CED-IADR 35th Annual Meeting September 23-25, 1999 Montpellier, France; *J. Dent. Res.*, 80:1194-255.

[5] Amat P 2003 May 2-6. Contribution of a functional and orthopaedic splint to the treatment of Class II malocclusions. 103rd Annual Session of the American Association of Orthodontists; Honolulu, Hawaii.

[6] Amat P. Apport d'une gouttière fonctionnelle et orthopédique au traitement des malocclusions de classe II. *Orthod. Fr.*, 2003;74:71-81.

[7] Amat P. Orthopédie dento-faciale fondée sur les faits : marotte d'universitaire ou indispensable outil clinique quotidien ? *Rev. Orthop. Dento. Faciale.*, 2006;40:421-51.

[8] Amat P. What would you choose: evidence-based treatment or an exciting, risky alternative? *Am. J. Orthod. Dentofacial. Orthop.*, 2007;132:724-5.

[9]   Amat P. Occlusion, orthodontics and posture: are there evidences? The example of scoliosis. *J. Stomat. Occ. Med.*, 2009;2: 2 – 10.
[10] Armijo Olivo S, Bravo J, Magee DJ, Thie NMR, Major PW, Flores-Mir C. The association between head and cervical posture and temporomandibular disorders: a systematic review. *J. Orofac. Pain.*, 2006;20:9–23.
[11] Bacon W, Turlot JC, Blaise M. La reproductibilité de la posture naturelle de la tête et son implication dans l'organisation de l'architecture craniofaciale. *Rev. Orthop. Dento.-Faciale.*, 1989;23:277-86.
[12] Ben-Bassat Y, Yitschaky M, Kaplan L, Brin I. Occlusal patterns in patients with idiopathic scoliosis. *Am. J. Orthod. Dentofacial. Orthop.*, 2006,130:629-33.
[13] Bodin CG, Duguet V, Hervé F. Diagnostic des latérognathies mandibulaires. Intérêt de la butée occlusale d'Abjean. Rev. Orthop. *Dento. Faciale.*, 1992;26:81-6.
[14] Bracco P, Deregibus A, Piscetta R, Ferrario G. Observations on the correlation between posture and jaw position: a pilot study. *Cranio*, 1998;16:252-8.
[15] Bracco P, Deregibus A, Piscetta R. Effects of different jaw relations on postural stability in human subjects.*Neurosci. Lett.*, 2004;356:228-30.
[16] Braun BL. Postural differences between asymptomatic men and women and craniofacial pain patients. *Arch. Phys. Med. Rehabil.*, 1991;72:653-6.
[17] Brenman HS. Amsterdam M. Postural effects on occlusion. *Dental Progress*, 1963;4:43-7.
[18] Browne PA, Clark GT, Kuboki T, Adachi NY. Concurrent cervical and craniofacial pain. A review of empiric and basic science evidence. *Oral Surg. Oral Med. Oral Pathol. Oral Radiol. Endod,* 1998;86:633-40.
[19] Burwell RG. Aetiology of idiopathic scoliosis: current concepts. *Pediatr. Rehabil.*, 2004;6:137-70.
[20] Campos AA, Nathanson D, Rose L. Reproducibility and condylar position of a physiologic maxillomandibular centric relation in upright and supine body position. *J. Prosthet. Dent.*, 1996;76:282-7.
[21] Commission de terminologie. Dictionnaire d'orthognathodontie. Paris. 2007. SFODF.
[22] Chapman RJ. et al. Occlusal contact variation with changes in head position. *Int. J. Prosthodont.*, 1991;4:377-81.
[23] Ciancaglini R. Proceedings of Research Forum. Posture, Occlusion and General Health.1997. Milan.

[24] Ciancaglini R. Proceedings of Research Forum. Posture and Occlusion: hypothesis of correlation, Consensus Conference ten years after. 2008. Milan.
[25] De Mayo T et al. Breathing type and body position effects on sternocleidomastoid and suprahyoid EMG activity. J Oral Rehabil 2005;32:487-94.
[26] D'Attilio M, Caputi S, Epifania E, Festa F, Tecco S. Evaluation of cervical posture of children in skeletal class I, II, and III. *Cranio*, 2005;23:219-28.
[27] D'Attilio M, Filippi M R, Femminella B, Festa F, Tecco S. The influence of an experimentally-induced malocclusion on vertebral alignment in rats: a controlled pilot study. *Journal of Craniomandibular Practice*, 2005;23:119-29.
[28] Deccache A. Quelles pratiques et compétences en éducation du patient ? Recommandations de l'O.M.S. *La Santé de l'homme*, 1999;341:12-4.
[29] Ferrario VF, Sforza C, Schmitz JH, Taroni A. Occlusion and center of foot pressure variation: is there a relationship? *J. Prosthet. Dent.*, 1996;76:302-8.
[30] Festa F, D'Attilio M, Vecchiet F. Effects of horizontal oscillation of the mandible on the spinal column of the rat in vivo using radiographic monitoring. *Ortogntodonzia. Ital.*, 1997;6:539-50.
[31] Festa F et al. Relationship between cervical lordosis and facial morphology in Caucasian women with a skeletal class II malocclusion: a cross-sectional study. *Cranio*, 2003;21:121-9.
[32] .Forgione AG, Mehta NR, Westcott WL. Strength and bite, Part 1: An analytical review. *Cranio*, 1991;9:305-15.
[33] Forgione AG, Mehta NR, McQuade CF, Westcott WL. Strength and bite, Part 2: Testing isometric strength using a MORA set to a functional criterion.*Cranio*, 1992;10:13-20.
[34] Gadotti IC, Bérzin F, Biasotto-Gonzalez D. Preliminary rapport on head posture and muscle activity in subjects with class I and II. *J. Oral. Rehabil.*, 2005;32:794-9.
[35] Gangloff P, Louis JP, Perrin PP. Dental occlusion modifies gaze and posture stabilization in human subjects. *Neurosci. Lett.*, 2000;293:203–6.
[36] Gangloff P, Perrin PP. Unilateral trigeminal anaesthesia modifies postural control in human subjects. *Neurosci. Lett.*, 2002;330:179–82
[37] Glenny AM, Harrison JE. How to interpret the orthodontic literature. *J. Orthod.*, 2003;30:159-64.

[38] Guillaumat M. Scoliose idiopathique de l'enfant et de l'adulte jeune. *Rev. Rhum.*, 2004;71:145-59.
[39] Hackney J, Bade D, Clawson A.Relationship between forward head posture and diagnosed internal derangement of the temporomandibular joint. *J. Orofac. Pain*, 1993;7:386-90.
[40] Hanke BA, Motschall E, Türp JC. Association between orthopedic and dental findings: what level of evidence is available? *J. Orofac. Orthop.*, 2007;68:91-107.
[41] Hellsing E, Hagberg C. Changes in maximum bite force related to extension of the head. *Eur. J. Orthod.*, 1990;12:148-53.
[42] Huggare J, Pirttiniemi P, Serlo W. Head posture and dentofacial morphology in subjects treated for scoliosis. *Proc. Finn. Dent. Soc.*, 1991;87:151-8.
[43] Huggare JA, Raustia AM. Head posture and cervicovertebral and craniofacial morphology in patients with craniomandibular dysfunction. *Cranio*, 1992;10:173-7.
[44] Ikemitsu H, Zeze R, Yuasa K, Izumi K. The relationship between jaw deformity and scoliosis. *Oral. Radiol.*, 2006;22:14–7.
[45] Komiyama O et al. Posture correction as part of behavioural therapy in treatment of myofascial pain with limited opening. *J. Oral. Rehabil.*, 1999;26:428-35.
[46] Kovero O et al. Maximal bite force and its associations with spinal posture and craniofacial morphology in young adults. *Acta. Odontol. Scand.*, 2002;60:365-9.
[47] Kritsineli M, Shim YS. Malocclusion, body posture, and temporomandibular disorder in children with primary and mixed dentition. *J. Clin. Pediatr. Dent.*, 1992;16:86-93.
[48] Lee WY, Okeson JP, Lindroth J.The relationship between forward head posture and temporomandibular disorders. *J. Orofac. Pain*, 1995;:161-7.
[49] LinksPersky SL, Johnston LE. An evaluation of dentofacial changes accompanying scoliosis therapy with a modified Milwaukee brace. *Am. J. Orthod.*, 1974;65 :364-71.
[50] Lippold C, van den Bos L, Hohoff A, Danesh G, Ehmer U. Interdisciplinary study of orthopedic and orthodontic findings in preschool infants. *J. Orofac. Orthop.*, 2003;64:330-40.
[51] Lonstein JE, Carlson JM. The prediction of curve progression in untreated idiopathic scoliosis during growth. *J. Bone Joint. Surg.*, 1984;66:1061–71.

[52] Makofsky HW. The influence of forward head posture on dental occlusion. *Cranio*, 2000;18:30-9.

[53] Mathis R, Bacon W, Siffert B. Facial growth of children wearing a modified Milwaukee brace. *Orthod. Fr.*, 1982;53:697-704.

[54] McLean LF, Brenman HS, Friedman MGF. Effects of changing body position on dental occlusion. *J. Dent. Res.*, 1973;52:1041-5.

[55] McNamara J, Seligman DA, Okeson JP. Occlusion, orthodontic treatment, and temporomandibular disorders: a review. *J. Orofacial. Pain*, 1995;9:73-90.

[56] Michelotti A et al. Postural stability and unilateral posterior crossbite: is there a relationship? *Neurosci. Lett.*, 2006;392:140-4.

[57] Michelotti A et al. Is unilateral posterior crossbite associated with leg length inequality? *Eur. J. Orthod.*, 2007;29:622-6.

[58] Miralles R et al. Body position effects on EMG activity of sternocleidomastoid and masseter muscles in healthy subjects.*Cranio*, 1998;16:90-9.

[59] Miralles R et al. Body position and jaw posture effects on supra- and infrahyoid electromyographic activity in humans.*Cranio*, 2006;24:98-103.

[60] Munhoz WC, Marques AP, de Siqueira JT. Evaluation of body posture in individuals with internal temporomandibular joint derangement. *Cranio*, 2005;23:269-77.

[61] Nobili A, Adversi R. Relationship between posture and occlusion: a clinical and experimental investigation. *Cranio*, 1996;14:274-85.

[62] Pećina M, Lulić-Dukić O, Pećina-Hrncević A. Hereditary orthodontic anomalies and idiopathic scoliosis. *Int. Orthop.*, 1991;15:57-9.

[63] Perinetti G. Dental occlusion and body posture: no detectable correlation. *Gait. Posture.*, 2006;24:165-8.

[64] Perinetti G. Temporomandibular disorders do not correlate with detectable alterations in body posture. *J. Contemp. Dent. Pract.*, 2007;8:60-7.

[65] Pollack B. Cases of note: Michigan jury awards $ 850,000 in ortho case: A tempest in a teapot. *Am. J. Orthod. Dentofacial. Orthop.*, 1988;94:358-9.

[66] Pradham NS, White GE, Mehta N, Forgione. A.Mandibular deviations in TMD and non-TMD groups related to eye dominance and head posture. *J. Clin. Pediatr. Dent.*, 2001;25:147-55.

[67] Roach JW. Adolescent idiopathic scoliosis. *Orthop. Clin. North. Am.*, 1999;30:353–65.

[68] Robin GC. The aetiology of idiopathic scoliosis. A review of a century of research. Boca Raton, 1990, Fla: Freund Publishing House.
[69] Roth NM. The modified monobloc appliance in scoliosis treatment. *Am. J. Orthod.*, 1969;55:506-9.
[70] Sackett D. Rules of evidence and clinical recommendations. *Can. J. Cardiol.*, 1993;9:487-9.
[71] Sackett DL, Rosenberg WM, Gray JA, Haynes RB, Richardson WS. Evidence based medicine: what it is and what it isn't. *BMJ* 1996;312:71-2.
[72] Saccucci et al.: Scoliosis and dental occlusion: a review of the literature. *Scoliosis*, 2011 6:15.
[73] Sakaguchi K et al. Examination of the relationship between mandibular position and body posture. *Cranio*, 2007;25:237-49.
[74] Salonen MA, Raustia AM, Huggare J . Head and cervical spine postures in complete denture wearers. *J. Craniomandib. Pract.*, 1993;11:30-3.
[75] Santander H et al. Influence of stabilisation occlusal splint on craniocervical relationships. Part II. electromyographic analysis. *J. Craniomandib. Pract.*, 1994;12:227-33.
[76] Santander H et al. Effects of head and neck inclination on bilateral sternocleidomastoid EMG activity in healthy subjects and in patients with myogenic cranio-cervical-mandibular dysfunction. *Cranio*, 2000;18:181-91.
[77] Slavicek R . Approche cybernétique des structures et fonctions de l'appareil manducateur. Communication aux IX Journées Internationales du CNO, in Actes des journées. 13, 14 et 15 mars 1992. Lyon.
[78] Solow B, Tallgren A . Dentoalveolar morphology in relation to craniocervical posture. *Angle. Orthod.*, 1977;47:157–64.
[79] Solow B, Sonnesen L. Head posture and malocclusions. *Eur. J. Orthod.*, 1998;20:685-93.
[80] Solow B, Sandham A. Cranio-cervical posture: a factor in the development and function of the dentofacial structures. *Eur. J. Orthod.*, 2002;24:447-56.
[81] Sonnesen L, Bakke M, Solow B. Temporomandibular disorders in relation to craniofacial dimensions, head posture and bite force in children selected for orthodontic treatment. *Eur. J. Orthod.*, 2001;23:179-92.
[82] Sonnesen L, Bakke M. Molar bite force in relation to occlusion, craniofacial dimensions, and head posture in pre-orthodontic children. *Eur. J. Orthod.*, 2005;27:58-63.

[83] Talmant J, Deniaud J. Optimal nasal ventilation: a physiological definition. *Arch. Pediatr.*, 2008;15:873-74.
[84] Tripodakis AP, Smulow JB, Mehta NR, Clark RE. Clinical study of location and reproducibility of three mandibular positions in relation to body posture and muscle function.*J. Prosthet. Dent.*, 1995;73:190-8.
[85] Valenzuela S et al. Does head posture have a significant effect on the hyoid bone position and sternocleidomastoid electromyographic activity in young adults? *Cranio*, 2005;23:204-11.
[86] Visscher CM, De Boer W, Lobbezoo F, Habets LL, Naeije M. Is there a relationship between head posture and craniomandibular pain? *J. Oral. Rehabil.*, 2002;29:1030-6.
[87] Vélez AL et al. Head posture and dental wear evaluation of bruxist children with primary teeth. *J. Oral. Rehabil.*, 2007;34:663-70.
[88] Weinstein SL, Buckwalter JA, editors. Turek's orthopedics, principles and their application. 5th ed. Philadelphia: 1994, JB Lippincott.
[89] Woda A, Pionchon P, Palla S. Regulation of mandibular postures: mechanisms and clinical implications. *Crit. Rev. Oral. Biol. Med.*, 2001;12:166-78.

In: Scoliosis: Causes, Symptoms and Treatment   ISBN: 978-1-62081-007-1
Editors: A. Bessette et al.   © 2012 Nova Science Publishers, Inc.

Chapter III

Shadow Moiré Technique to Measure Deformity of the Trunk Surface in the Elderly: A Population-based Study

Flávia Porto[1,2,4,*], *Jonas Lírio Gurgel*[2],
Thais Russomano[3] *and Paulo de Tarso Veras Farinatti*[4]

[1]Stricto Sensu Post Graduation in Exercise Science and Sports,
Gama Filho University, Brazil
[2]Biomechanics Research Group, Institute of Physical Education,
Fluminense Federal University, Brazil
[3]Microgravity Centre, School of Engineering, Pontifical Catholic
University of Rio Grande do Sul, Brazil
[4]Physical Activity and Health Promotion Laboratory, Institute of Physical
Education and Sports, Rio de Janeiro State University, Brazil

---

[*] Correspondence to: Flávia Porto, PhD. Programa de Pós-graduação Stricto Sensu em Ciências do Exercício e do Esporte, PPGEF, UGF. Rua Manoel Vitorino, 553 - Prédio AG 5° andar. Bairro Piedade.
C.E.P.: 20748-900 Rio de Janeiro – RJ – Brasil. Telephone: (55xx21) 2599 7138; E-mail address: flavia_porto@msn.com/ flaviaporto_@terra.com.br.

Abstract

Since 1970, the Moiré phenomenon has been employed as a method of clinical diagnosis in topographical analyses of the human body. This study aimed to evaluate the trunk posture of the elderly population in South Brazil using Shadow Moiré Technique (SMT). This is a cross-sectional, observational, exploratory and randomized study. SMT was applied to people over 60 years (n= 444; 331 women and 113 men) living in Porto Alegre-RS, Brazil. Lateral deviations of the thoracic spine, the alignment of scapula in the frontal and transverse planes, and the depth of torso were assessed. The data was presented as mean, standard deviation and percentiles (P5, P10, P25, P50, P75, P90, P95). Age and gender differences were tested using 2-way ANOVA followed by the Bonferroni post-hoc test whenever indicated (p ≤ 0.05). The results for men showed a reduction in scapular alignment with progressive age, whereas this commenced in women only from 80 years of age. In relation to gender differences, men and women showed similarities in this variable for all ages. Thoracic kyphosis showed increases with age for men and women, and no statistical differences were found between genders. The age group 60-69 years showed statistical differences on right side gibosity (p=0.002), whilst for the left side, there were gender differences for the 60-69 years (p=0.000) and 70-79 years (p=0.016) age groups. There was no relationship between: the scapular alignment on frontal plane and angular spine variation on frontal plane; alignment between scapulas on transverse plane and angular spine variation on frontal plane of men and women. The results showed that SMT was useful for the evaluation of trunk deformities in the elderly.

Keywords: Moiré Topography; Aged; Posture

Introduction

Postural deviations become worse with age due to a combination of factors such as the onset of osteoporosis [1], degeneration of intervertebral discs [2] (Zhao et al., 2007), weakness of musculoskeletal system [3], and accumulated vertebral fractures, especially in frail elderly people [4]. The aging process is associated with spine changes in the sagittal plane, reflecting on vertebral segments and posture [5]. Discomfort caused by postural deviations may impact on the ability to perform daily living activities, therefore jeopardizing autonomy and quality of life [6].

Hence, posture evaluation would seem to be an important aspect of health promotion throughout aging. Prior knowledge of potential postural deviations may help in the design of specific rehabilitation programs for the elderly [7, 8]. From a broader perspective, population-based studies are thought to provide more general epidemiologic data on the profile of postural deviations in a given cohort, which can help when determining their probable cause and developing prevention strategies [9]. Such population-based studies are accessible for many different countries [10], but unfortunately data concerning the Brazilian population in particular is scarce.

This is problematic as the elderly population of Brazil is increasing. The number of citizens aged 60 years and above reached 21 million in 2009 and it is estimated that by 2050, they will make up 30% of the total population [11]. The average life expectancy of Brazilians increased from 45.5 years in 1940 to 72.7 years in 2008, meaning an additional 27.2 years of life. According to official projections [12], this figure will continue to increase and will reach 81.3 years by 2050, nearly equaling the current figures for Iceland (81.8 years) and Japan (82.6 years). Therefore, conducting further population-based studies on the postural characteristics of the elderly in Brazil would be useful.

The Shadow Moiré Technique (SMT) is a non-invasive optical technique that may be used for the detection and follow up of spinal deformities, such as scoliosis [13]. Moiré topography has been used to assess the posture of young people in the detection of deformations of the trunk [14-16]. This topographic method is low-cost and radiation free, enabling many subjects to be evaluated over a short time period [16]. The SMT technique can, in fact, replace assessment via X-ray and is acknowledged as a complementary method for upper body deformity diagnosis [15, 17, 18]. The procedure does not require highly trained professionals for its application [16, 19], and previous studies have demonstrated that the method is easily reproducible. The technique has already been used as a tool for qualitative diagnosis [15, 16].

However, there appears to be a lack of population-based studies using this technique, particularly in elderly populations [20, 21]. One of the possible limiting factors for the use of this technique in epidemiologic studies may be the fatigue associated with the manual visual inspection of the Moiré fringes [20], which can lead to misinterpretation. A more widespread use of SMT may occur when the task of interpreting the topograms has become automated. Development of automated strategies for analyzing the Moiré patterns would increase the potential application of the SMT in population-based research [16, 20, 22].

Thus, the present study aimed to assess trunk postural deviations in the frontal, sagittal and transverse planes using the SMT, in a cohort of men and women aged 60 years and above living in the city of Porto Alegre (southern Brazil). Additionally, the use of a free-software to analyze the Moiré topograms has been tested and validated.

Methods

Subjects

The strategies previously employed by the Multidimensional Study of Living Conditions of the Elderly [23] were used for sample selection. Initially, 64 households with older residents were randomly selected and stratified proportionally according to the last official census for the city of Porto Alegre [24]. The data was assessed in two phases between December 2005 and September 2006. In the first phase, 1,164 subjects were interviewed by social service professionals about epidemiologic indicators related to housing, family composition, social relations, occupation, income, socio-cultural aspects, sexuality, aging, health, and activities of daily living. In the second phase, the same elderly people were invited to participate in a large and interdisciplinary assessment (Architecture and Urbanism, Physical Education, Nursing, Pharmacy, Physical Therapy, Geriatrics, Nutrition, and Psychology).

Only the subjects who accepted and attended the second phase participated in the SMT analysis. However, those who were unable to stand for the photos were excluded. This resulted in a final sample figure of 331 women and 113 men (60-89 years old), to whom the SMT analysis was applied.

The present study is part of a Multidimensional Study of the Elderly in Porto Alegre (MSEPOA), which was approved by institutional Ethics and Research Committee (Approval No. 1.066/05-CEP). The volunteers were informed about the investigation and signed a consent form authorizing disclosure of their data for research.

Shadow Moiré Technique Assessment

The SMT assessment was performed using a specific setup including a) Moiré reticulum (grid), with intervals of 1mm x 1mm, made with nylon threads; b) Digital photographic camera (Brand Canon, Model 7i, Sao Paulo,

Brazil); Tripod; Light source of 100W. The SMT arrangement is illustrated in the Figure 1.

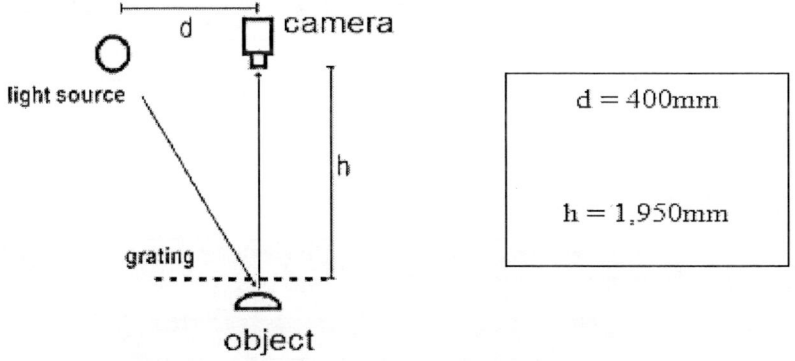

Figure 1. Setup for the application of SMT for postural analysis.

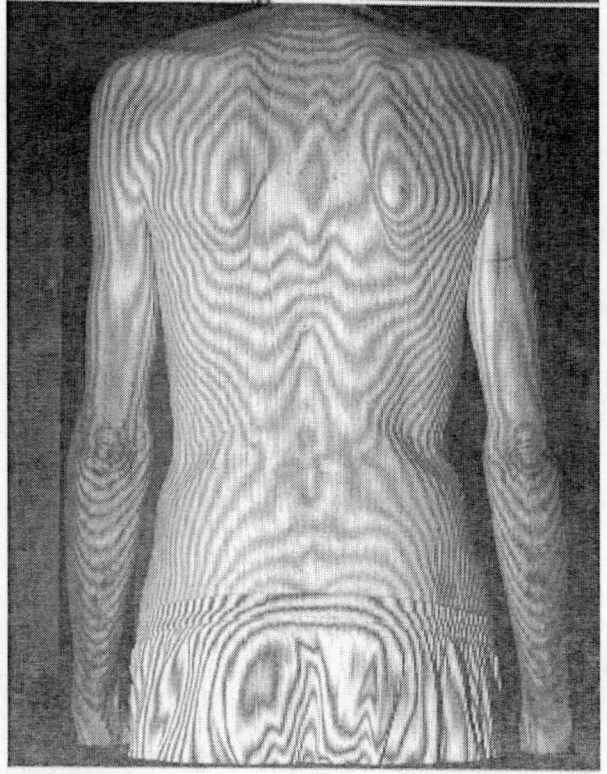

Figure 2. Moiré topogram [25].

Table 1. Anthropometric variables in the elderly assessed with SMT

	Age group	n	Mean	SD	Percentile					
					5	10	25	50	75	90	95
Men											
Body mass (kg)	60-69	55	78.7	16.3	55.3	57.7	64.1	78.0	89.5	101.9	110.8
	70-79	45	75.4	16.7	51.2	54.4	65.7	71.3	84.4	96.2	107.9
	80-89	12	68.2	8.5	55.3	55.5	59.3	70.6	75.9	78.7	79.4
Height (cm)	60-69	55	168.8	7.5	155.3	159.2	163.7	169.3	174.7	179.0	179.2
	70-79	46	166.4	6.8	153.6	157.2	161.9	165.8	170.7	174.6	179.5
	80-89	12	165.9	5.8	158.0	158.4	161.5	165.7	168.7	177.2	179.5
Women											
Body mass (kg)	60-69	153	72	16.9	50.7	54.2	60.5	69.5	80.3	88.6	99.2
	70-79	102	68.4	13.7	46.6	51.3	59.4	68.5	75.6	85.5	94.3
	80-89	40	57.8	11.2	41.4	44.5	49.3	56.9	65.2	74.5	82.4
Height (cm)	60-69	154	154.8	6.3	143.2	146.4	150.2	155.3	159.5	162.5	164.1
	70-79	103	152.5	9.8	143.1	145.0	148.5	153.0	157.5	162.3	165.1
	80-89	40	150.6	6.6	140.1	141.9	144.7	151.3	155.0	160.5	161.8
	90+	3	151.2	4.8	148.3	148.3	148.5	156.7	156.7	156.7

SD = Standard Deviation.
n = sample size.

The equipment was calibrated prior to the assessment [17] and the room darkened with black cloth and lights turned off. The subjects remained barefoot during the test, with their backs exposed and were placed behind the grid in a standing position. The back was towards the grid and situated as close as possible without actually touching it. Two images of the back were obtained, with 256 shades of grey, ranging from 0 (black) to 255 (white) (Figure 2).

The topogram analysis was performed using the free-software Power Draw 2D (Vector Application, Tekhnelogos, Istanbul, Turkey). Lateral deviations of the thoracic spine, the alignment of scapula in the frontal and transverse planes, and the depth of torso were assessed. In order to check for the presence of thoracic hyperkyphosis, the number of fringes that appeared from the centroid scapulars to C7 were counted, and the result inserted in a specific equation to calculate the depth of the fringes [18, 26, 27].

Statistical and Qualitative Analyses

The subjects were stratified into three age groups (60-69, 70-79 and 80-89 years). Data normality was confirmed by univariate analysis. Anthropometric characteristics (body mass and height) were presented as mean, standard deviation and percentiles (P5, P10, P25, P50, P75, P90, P95). Similar descriptive statistics were also presented for the alignment of both scapula in the frontal and transverse planes, and for anteroposterior deviations of the thoracic column. Lateral deviations of the spine were classified according to the identified concavities (concave to the right or left, and concave-convex to the right or left) and showed as histograms. Age and gender differences were tested using 2-way ANOVA followed by the Bonferroni post-hoc test whenever indicated (p ≤ 0.05). All calculations were performed using the software SPSS 11.5 for Windows (SPSS, New York, USA).

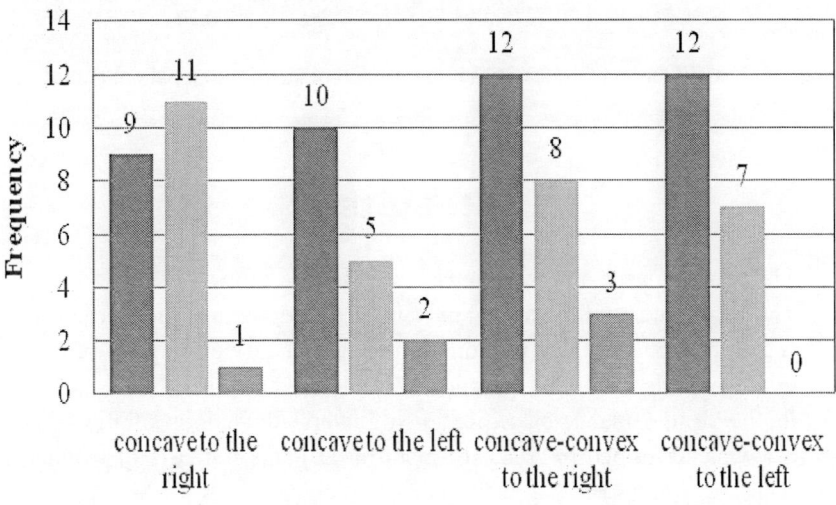

Figure 3. Classification of concavities in the frontal plane of the spinal column of men.

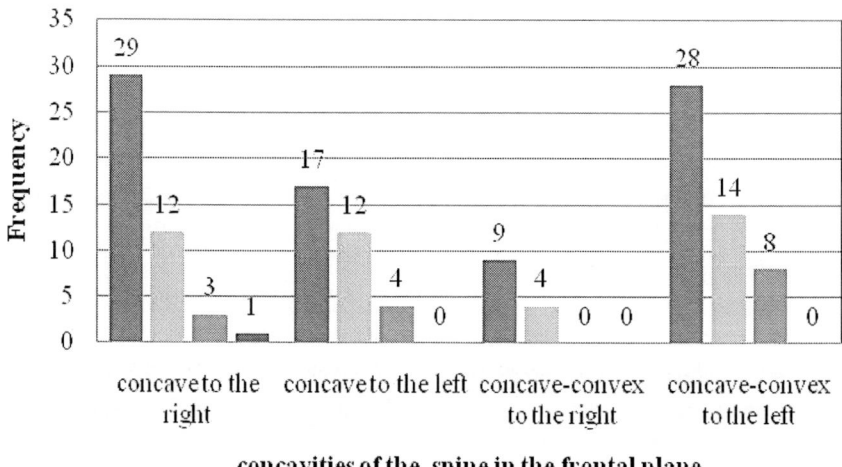

Figure 4. Classification of concavities in the frontal plane of the spinal column of women.

Results

The results for the anthropometric variables are showed in Table 1.

The technique employed for analysis of the topograms did not permit all subjects to be evaluated due to limitations in the quality of photographs and/or due to the large deformity of the trunk presented by the individual.

In the frontal plane, classification of lateral deviations of the spine in subjects was performed in 70.8% of men (n= 80) and in 42.6% of women (n= 141) (Figures 3 and 4).

Analysis of the scapulas in the frontal plane using the procedure of Moiré topograms could be made in 75.2% of men studied (n=85) and in 55.9% of women (n=185) (Table 2).

The evaluation of anterior-posterior thoracic curvature could be accomplished in 100% of the sample (n=444) (Table 3).

In the transverse plane, the alignment of the scapular region was evaluated, with the results demonstrating the presence of a gibbus in 77.9% of men (n=88) and in 82.8% of women (n=274) (Table 4).

Table 2. Descriptive results (mean, standard deviation and percentile, in degree) of alignment of the scapulas in the frontal plane of the elderly in Porto Alegre

	Age Group (years)	n	Mean (degree)	SD (degree)	Percentile (degree)					
					5	10	25	50	75	90	95
Men	60-69	45	0.2	6.0	-9.00	-7.4	-4.0	0.0	3.0	6.0	10.2
	70-79	36	0.7	5.2	-8.2	-5.3	-3.0	.50	4.0	8.3	10.3
	80-89	4	2.3	3.6	-1.0	-1.0	-0.8	1.5	6.0	7.0	7.0
Women	60-69	105	0.9	5.8	-9.7	-6.4	-3.0	0.0	4.5	8.4	9.0
	70-79	58	-0.7	5.2	-11.0	-10.1	-4.0	-0.5	3.00	6.0	8.0
	80-89	21	-1.2	6.7	-20.5	-6.6	-5.0	-3.0	3.5	7.0	8.8

SD = Standard Deviation.
n = sample size.

Table 3. Descriptive results of anteroposterior deviations (mm) of the thoracic column in the elderly of Porto Alegre

	Age Group (years)	N	Mean (mm)	SD (mm)	Percentile (mm)					
					5	10	25	50	75	90	95
Men	60-69	55	38.1	19.2	0.0	0.0	29.7	39.8	50.0	65.5	66.5
	70-79	46	43.9	22.2	1.7	19.7	29.7	42.3	55.1	70.7	84.7
	80-89	12	44.7	21.2	0.0	8.9	31.0	42.3	55.1	78.1	81.3
Women	60-69	170	39.8	21.5	0.0	10.3	29.7	39.8	50.0	65.5	76.0
	70-79	114	42.5	24.0	0.0	0.0	29.7	39.8	55.1	68.1	97.2
	80-89	43	42.6	24.7	0.0	0.0	29.7	39.8	60.3	68.6	88.7

SD = Standard Deviation.
n = sample size.

Gender Influence

When comparing the values of alignment between the scapulas in the frontal plane, there were no statistically significant differences encountered between genders in the age groups 60-69 years ($p = 0.361$), 70-79 years ($p = 0.205$) and 80-89 years ($p = 0.324$).

In regards to the alignment of the scapulas in the transverse plane, the right and left scapular regions of the individuals were compared with respect to the depth of the areas. When comparing genders, for the right side, the results illustrated significant differences in the age group 60-69 years ($p = 0.002$), but not between 70-79 years ($p = 0.412$) and 80-89 years ($p = 0.308$).

For the left side, the results showed statistical differences in the age groups 60-69 years (p < 0.001) and 70-79 years (p = 0.016), unlike in the age group 80-89 years (p = 0.065).

With reference to the kyphotic thoracic arch, the results showed that there were no statistically significant differences between men and women in the age group 60-69 years (p = 0.901), 70-79 years (p = 0.813) and 80-89 years (p = 0.791).

Table 4. Descriptive results of scapular alignment in the transverse plane of the elderly in Porto Alegre

	Age Group	n	Mean	SD	Percentile						
					5	10	25	50	75	90	95
Men											
N° of centroids on right side	60-69	44	2.8[a]	1.4	1.0	1.0	2.0	3.0	4.0	5.0	5.0
	70-79	37	2.0[a]	1.5	0.0	0.0	1.0	2.0	3.0	4.0	4.3
	80-89	4	1.8	0.5	1.0	1.0	1.3	2.0	2.0	2.0	2.0
	70-79	39	2.3	1.4	1.0	1.0	1.0	2.0	3.0	4.0	5.0
	80-89	4	2.0	0.8	1.0	1.0	1.3	2.0	2.8	3.0	3.0
Women											
N° of centroids on right side	60-69[b]	146	2.1	1.3	0.0	0.0	1.0	2.0	3.0	4.0	4.7
	70-79	93	1.8	1.4	0.0	0.0	1.0	2.0	2.5	4.0	4.0
	80-89[b]	33	1.4	0.9	0.0	0.0	1.0	1.0	2.0	2.6	3.0
	90+	2	2.0	1.4	1.0	1.0	1.0	2.0	3.0	3.0	3.0
N° of centroids on left side	60-69[c]	146	1.7	1.1	0.0	0.0	1.0	1.5	2.0	3.0	4.0
	70-79	93	1.6	0.9	0.0	1.0	1.0	2.0	2.0	3.0	3.0
	80-89[c]	33	1.1	0.9	0.0	0.0	0.5	1.0	2.0	2.6	3.0

SD = Standard Deviation.
n = sample size.
[a]p=0.043; [b]p=0.017; [c]p=0.019.

Discussion

This study aimed to investigate with the use of SMT, postural deviations of the trunk observed in the frontal, sagittal and transversal planes, of people over the age of 60 living in the city of Porto Alegre, Brazil, linking it to gender and age group differences. The major findings were: a) the angular spine variation of men in the frontal plane was higher in the 60-69 years group; b) this angular spine variation in women presented a tendency to decrease until 79 years, and increasing from 80 years. Other than this, the data showed no statistical differences between genders for postural deviations in the frontal plane; c) the men showed a reduction in scapular alignment with progressive aging, whilst with women this started only at 80 years. In relation to gender, men and women showed similarities in this variable for all ages; d) thoracic kyphosis showed increases with aging for both men and women and no statistical difference was found between genders. The age group 60-69 years showed statistical differences for right side gibosity (p=0.002), whilst for the left side, there were gender differences for the 60-69 years (p=0.000) and 70-79 years (p=0.016) age groups; e) the thoracic kyphosis increases with aging for both genders and showed no significant differences between age groups.

Since Takasaki [18, 26, 28] demonstrated the various applications for the Moiré phenomenon, especially in the clinical area, SMT has begun to be used in the detection of spinal deformities [15-17, 19, 22, 27, 29, 30].

The technique employed for the analyses of the Moiré topograms in this study has been used previously [17, 30]. It was not possible to assess all of the individuals for all of the pre-established variables using the proposed image analysis technique, other than for the depth of kyphotic thoracic curvature. Despite this, it did permit the detection of postural alterations in the three orthogonal planes. Perhaps the body shape of the subject is a restrictive aspect for the use of this technique, since it is based on the inspection of the body surface.

Authors [29, 31] confirm the use of Moiré Topography (MT) for the precise determination of characteristics, such as length, depth and angulation of body surfaces. Additionally, these studies have shown a correlation with the x-ray results [32, 33], making the SMT a useful complementary diagnostic tool.

Some authors consider that difficulties in generating good quality topograms can be related to the control of intervening variables in the SMT process, and this, consequently, may interfere with the accuracy of measurements. These complications can be attributed to the translucent nature of the skin being evaluated, the accuracy of the grid construction, and the care taken when applying the test, such as making sure the individual does not move while the image is taken during the examination [27]. In this study, we sought to minimize the errors of interpretation of the Moiré patterns during the postural exam through standardizing the placement of volunteers for the test and also by the use of trained assessors for the exam, according to guidelines in the literature [34].

The results of this study indicated some degree of lateral deviation of the spine in participants of both sexes. Authors [19] confirmed that MT can also detect these two types of scoliosis. The classification of scoliosis using SMT, is based primarily on the asymmetry of the Moiré fringes projected onto the back of the individual [27]. The diagnosis of scoliosis by the use of Moiré is very variable in the scientific literature. A lack of standardization in assessment procedures and of equipment used can be seen, making it difficult to compare the results of this study with those obtained by other authors. Additionally, the profile of subjects evaluated in this study (the elderly) differs from the subject profile commonly considered in most scientific studies surveyed (children and adolescents).

When considering the analysis of Moiré topograms for the scapula region, researchers [35] claim that despite the differences in images of the back from person to person, there are many common characteristics. It is noted that the fringes in the area of the scapular cavity are concentric curves - called centroids. The center of the scapula cavity can be characterized as the center of the fringe inherent to that area. This principle was also one of the variables adopted by Chalupova [36] in her study modeling biomechanics of the scapulas using SMT, and in other studies on postural evaluation [17, 30].

While there is an in-built error in considering the center of gravity (COG) of a quadrilateral tracing around the centroids as being equivalent to the COG of the respective centroid, inasmuch as sometimes these COG's do not visually match, this was also an evaluation procedure for topograms used by other authors [17, 30, 37]. Moreover, considering that the COG of an object refers to the virtual point at which its mass is uniformly distributed, it is assumed that the COG will be located where more mass is distributed [38].

The fact that each centroid or Moiré fringe is characterized as a level curve, it is assumed that the more fringes present in a particular area, the deeper it is. In this way, the accentuated curves, when comparing the right and left sides, can be due to the presence of a gibbus on the back of the individual [19, 37].

The alignment of the scapulas can interfere with the developed function of the shoulders, and therefore the upper limbs. The loss of this function in the elderly has been the subject of study by some authors [39].

The results relating to the analysis of thoracic kyphosis showed that men strayed from the midline of the body, approximately 40mm to the front (flexion) in the age group 60-69, and up to ± 50mm in the group 80-89 years. In the female group aged 90, the depth could be greater than ± 60mm. These values are significant bearing in mind that the measurement was taken from the scapular region and taking into consideration how much the vertebral segment had moved away from the midline of the body.

The incidence of thoracic hyperkyphosis was measured on the premise that the points belonging to the same fringe have the same height, and the difference between the neighbouring parallel Moiré fringes is relatively constant [18, 35]. The fact that we found significant curvature in this region of the vertebral column deserves attention and corroborates the point that older people, in fact, present a hyperkyphotic profile when compared to younger individuals [3, 5, 40, 41].

Recent studies have discussed the relationship between pronounced kyphotic curvature of elderly people, the presence of vertebral osteoporosis, and the influence of these factors on subject quality of life. Weakening and deterioration in the quality of bone tissue can lead to a series of small fractures. After the first vertebral fracture, the risk of a subsequent fracture increases significantly ('vertebral fracture cascade phenomenon'). These fractures can cause increased kyphotic curvature in the physiology of the individual and affect neurophysiological properties related principally to the control of equilibrium and mobility of the torso [4]. This instability of postural balance may be due to a fracture in a specific location in the column, rather than the number of fractures presented and the consequent deformity of the vertebral column that this leads to [42].

It is important to stress that in the case of a topographic method, SMT covers all the surface area being evaluated. Therefore, one must consider that in addition to bone deformities that can be seen on the body surface, other factors can contribute to the analysis results. For that matter, edema, excess skin or hair, and eczema are also factors that can interfere. X-ray examination would be the ideal alternative if requiring detailed diagnosis of an individual's bone structure, along with other tests such as bone densitometry.

It was suggested in this study that SMT be used as a complementary method for postural evaluation. Also presented was percentile data about the variables studied. These become relevant measures in that the percentiles translate into comparable variables. For example, to say that a senior citizen of 70 years has a thoracic kyphosis depth value of 5mm does not mean much on its own, but by comparing this value with the measures presented by the elderly population, we can say that this elderly person has a greater degree of curvature than 50% of the population in that age group. Percentiles are used in the control of athletes' training, and were used in the description of parameters researched for population studies of the elderly [43, 44].

The postural profile of a person gives much relevant information about their physical health and appearance. Postural assessment can serve as a method of complementary evaluation providing a cross-referenced and more conclusive understanding of health aspects of the elderly.

Study Limitations

Some limitations were identified during this study. The voluntary population-based research brought some consequences such as non-attendance of some selected subjects in Phase 1 of MSEPOA. The use of SMT in the study was also a limiting factor as no standardized testing procedures appeared in the literature. Additionally, the lack of research using this technique with an elderly population prevented comparison of the results with similar studies. Moreover, the non-automated process was a factor that hindered the analyses of some images.

Acknowledgments

The authors are grateful to the Scholarship Program to Support Graduate Private Education Institutions (PROSUP/ CAPES/ BRAZIL).

Conclusion

Signs of scoliosis in "S" form were more present in younger men, while women of the same age group presented deformities in "C" form. Differences in alignment of the scapula in the frontal plane were less than 1 degree for both genders, in most age groups. In the transverse plane, the presence of a gibbus was detected in most individuals. In the sagittal plane, the anterior-posterior thoracic curvature increased with the progression of age for all individuals. Statistical differences in regards to gender were found only in the alignment between the scapulas in the transverse plane. The SMT proved to be useful for the assessment of trunk deformities of the elderly in Porto Alegre, Brazil. The study suggests that use of the technique can be applied in the elderly leading to good results for evidence of deformities of the trunk. This widens the application possibilities of the technique, which has historically been used to assess young people.

References

[1] Granito R. *Effects of aging and osteoporosis in thoracic kyphosis in proprioception and trunk muscle torque.* São Carlos, SP: Universidade Federal de São Carlos; 2005.

[2] Zhao CQ, Wang LM, Jiang LS, Dai LY. The cell biology of intervertebral disc aging and degeneration. *Ageing research reviews.* 2007 Oct;6(3):247-61.

[3] Hinman M. Comparison of thoracic kyphosis and postural stiffness in younger and older women. *The Spine Journal.* 2004;4(4):413-7.

[4] Brigs A, Greig A, Wark J. The vertebral fracture cascade in osteoporosis: a review of aetiopathogenesis. *Osteoporos Int.* 2007;18:575-84.

[5] Salter R. *Distúrbios e lesões do sistema musculoesquelético.* Rio de Janeiro: MEDSI 2001.

[6] Takahashi T, Ishida K, Hirose D, Nagano Y, Okumiya K, Nishinaga M, Matsubayashi K, Doi Y, Tani T, Yamamoto H. Trunk deformity is associated with a reduction in outdoor activities of daily living and life satisfaction in community-dwelling older people. *Osteoporos Int.* 2005 16:273-9.

[7] Sinaki M. Exercise and osteoporosis. *Arch Phys Med Rehabil.* 1989 Mar;70(3):220-9.

[8] Burke TN, Franca FJ, Ferreira de Meneses SR, Cardoso VI, Marques AP. Postural control in elderly persons with osteoporosis: Efficacy of an intervention program to improve balance and muscle strength: a randomized controlled trial. American journal of physical medicine & rehabilitation/*Association of Academic Physiatrists.* 2010 Jul;89(7):549-56.

[9] Jaovisidha S, Kim JK, Sartoris DJ, Bosch E, Edelstein S, Barrett-Connor E, Rojanaplakorn P. Scoliosis in elderly and age-related bone loss: a population-based study. *J Clin Densitom.* 1998 Fall;1(3):227-33.

[10] Chaiwanichsiri D, Jiamworakul A, Jitapunkul S. Lumbar disc degeneration in Thai elderly: a population-based study. *Journal of the Medical Association of Thailand = Chotmaihet thangphaet.* 2007 Nov;90(11):2477-81.

[11] Carvalho JAMd, Rodríguez-Wong LL. The changing age distribution of the Brazilian population in the fi rst half of the 21st century. *Cad Saúde Pública.* 2008;24(3):597-605.

[12] Brazilian Institute of Geography and Statistics – IBGE. *2010 Census*. 2010. [captured in: 2011 Apr 04]. Available in: http://www.ibge.gov.br/
[13] Moran AJ, Lipczynski RT. Automatic digitization and analysis of moire topograms on a personal computer for clinical use. *Medical engineering & physics*. 1994 May;16(3):259-64.
[14] Kovac V, Pecina M. Moire topography in measurement of the sagittal curvatures of the spine. *Coll Antropol*. 1999 Jun;23(1):153-8.
[15] Adler N, Csongradi J, Bleck E. School screening for scoliosis – one experience in California using clinical examination and Moiré Photography. *West J Med*. 1984;141(5):631-3.
[16] Yeras A, Peña R, Junco R. Moiré topography: alternative technique in health care. *Opt Lasers Eng*. 2003;40:105-16.
[17] Hertz H, Russomano T, Porto F, Gurgel J, Steiger A, Azevedo D. Development of the Shadow Moiré technique as a low cost alternative to postural analysis. Scientia Medica. 2005;15:235-42.
[18] Takasaki H. Moiré Topography. *Appl Opt*. 1970;9(6):1467-72.
[19] Batouche M, Benlamri R. A computer vision system for diagnosing scoliosis. In: IEEE, ed. *IEEE International Conference on Pervasive Computing and Communications*. Orlando, Florida 1994:2623-28.
[20] Kim H, Ishikawa S, Ohtsuka Y, Shimizu H, Shinomiya T, Viergever M. Automatic scoliosis detection based on local centroids evaluation on Moiré topographic images of human backs. *IEEE Trans Med Imaging*. 2001;20(12):1314-20.
[21] Lim JS, Kim J, Chung MS. Automatic shadow moire topography: a moving-light-source method. *Opt Lett*. 1989 November 15;14(22):1252-3.
[22] Kim H, Tan J, Ishikawa S, Khalid M, Otsuka Y, Shimizu H, Shinomiya T. Automatic judgment of spinal deformity based on back propagation on neural network. *IJICIC*. 2006;2(6):1271-9.
[23] Bós A, Bós A. Determinants of elders choice between private and public health care providers. *Rev Saúde Pública* [Electronic Article]. 2004 [capturado 2007 Nov 6]; 38 (1): Disponível em: http://www.scielo.br/scielo.php?pid=S0034-89102004000100016&script=sci_arttext&tlng=pt#back1
[24] Brazilian Institute of Geography and Statistics. *Perfil dos idosos responsáveis por domicílios no Brasil* 2000. Rio de Janeiro: IBGE 2002.
[25] Porto F, Gurgel JL, Farinatti PdTV. Moiré topography as a method of postural evaluation: state of the art review. *Brazilian Journal of Geriatrics and Gerontology* 2011.

[26] Takasaki H. Simultaneous all-around measurement of a living body by Moiré topography. *Congress of the International Society of Photogrammetry*. Helsinki 1976:1527-34.
[27] Takasaki H. Moiré topography from its birth to practical application. *Opt Lasers Eng.* 1982;3:3-14.
[28] Takasaki H. Moire Topography. *Appl Opt.* 1973;12(4):845-50.
[29] Batouche M. A knowledge based system for diagnosing apinal deformations: Moiré pattern analysis and interpretation. *11th IAPR International Conference on Pattern Recognition*: Conference A: Computer Vision and Applications, *IEEE Trans Med Imaging* 1992: 591-4.
[30] Hertz H. *Construction of the calibration technique for analysis of shadow moiré postural [monograph]*. Porto Alegre: Pontifical Catholic University of Rio Grande do Sul; 2005.
[31] Przysada G, Pop T, Kolodziej K, Rusek W. Application of Moire's method for posture evaluation in patients with low back pain syndrome. *ADREH.* 2005(1):103-7.
[32] Daruwalla J, Balasubramaniam P. Moiré topography in scoliosis: its accuracy in detecting the site and size of the curve. *J Bone Joint Surg.* 1985;67-B(2):211-3.
[33] Pearsall D, Reid J, Hedden D. Comparison of three noninvasive methods for measuring scoliosis. *Phys Ther.* 1992;72(9):648-57.
[34] Drerup B. A procedure for the numerical analysis of Moiré topograms. *Photogramm.* 1981;36:41-9.
[35] Batouche M, Benlamri R, Kholladi M. A computer vision system for diagnosing scoliosis using Moiré images. *Comput Biol Med.* 1996;26(4):339-53.
[36] Chalupová M. *Use of a biomechanical model of the scapula region for the identification of muscle disbalance*. [Electronic Article]. 2001 [capturado 2005 Jul 30]; Disponível em: mms.tudelft.nl/dsg/intersg /Proceedings_2001_files/06_chalupova.pdf
[37] Mínguez M, Buendía M, Cibrián R, Salvador R, Laguía M, Martín A, Gomar F. Quantifier variables of the back surface deformity obtained with a noninvasive structured light method: evaluation of their usefulness in idiopathic scoliosis diagnosis. *Eur Spine J.* 2007;16:73–82.
[38] Enoka R. *Neuromechanics of human movement.* 3 ed. Champaign, IL: Human Kinetics 2001.

[39] Abizanda P, Navarro JL, Romero L, Leon M, Sanchez-Jurado PM, Dominguez L. Upper extremity function, an independent predictor of adverse events in hospitalized elderly. *Gerontology*. 2007;53(5):267-73.
[40] Oliveira L. *Osteoporose: guia para diagnóstico, prevenção e tratamento*. Rio de Janeiro: Revinter 2002.
[41] Spirduso W. *Dimensões físicas do envelhecimento*. São Paulo: Manole 2005.
[42] Greig A, Bennell K, Briggs A, Wark J, Hodges P. Balance impairment is related to vertebral fracture rather than thoracic kyphosis in individuals. *Osteoporos Int*. 2007;18:543-51.
[43] Santos JL, Albala C, Lera L, Garcia C, Arroyo P, Perez-Bravo F, Angel B, Pelaez M. Anthropometric measurements in the elderly population of Santiago, Chile. *Nutrition*. 2004 May;20(5):452-7.
[44] Suriah A, Zalifah M, Zainorni M, Shafawi S, Mimie Suraya S, Zarina N, Wan Zainuddin W. Anthropometric measurements of the elderly. *Mal J Nutr* 1998;4:55-63.

In: Scoliosis: Causes, Symptoms and Treatment   ISBN: 978-1-62081-007-1
Editors: A. Bessette et al.   © 2012 Nova Science Publishers, Inc.

Chapter IV

Scoliosis: Causes, Symptoms and Treatment

Reuben C.C. Soh[1] and Hwan Tak Hee[2]
[1] Department of Orthopaedic Surgery,
KK Women's and Children's Hospital, Singapore
[2] Centre for Spine & Scoliosis Surgery, Singapore
Mount Elizabeth Medical Centre, Singapore

Abstract

Scoliosis remains a common problem faced by orthopaedists and pediatricians worldwide. Current epidemiological studies place the prevalence of scoliosis at 3% in the general population. The commonest type of scoliosis is adolescent idiopathic scoliosis. To date, there have been many theories but no proven direct cause of idiopathic scoliosis. Genetics, central nervous factors, collagen, muscle and platelet defects, hormonal factors, as well as biomechanical factors seem to play a role in the development of this deformity.

Adolescents seldom complain of pain and often the first presentation to the orthopedist is following a referral from the primary care physician or a school screening program. The confirmation of scoliosis follows a radiograph showing at least 10 degrees of coronal deformity in the standing scoliosis x-ray. Back pain and pulmonary complications are rare in scoliosis except when the curve is severe. These problems are more pronounced in the infantile and juvenile scoliosis, often due to the rapid progression of the Cobb angle.

Treatment is targeted at prevention of worsening deformity, and thus hopefully preventing the need for surgical intervention. A conservative approach is undertaken with the use of rigid or dynamic bracing which is carried out until skeletal maturity. The success of bracing with congenital scoliosis is limited and many will require surgical intervention eventually.

Surgical intervention of scoliosis involve posterior instrumentation and fusion in skeletally mature individuals and the use of non-fusion procedures such as growing rods and vertical expandable prosthetic titanium rib (VEPTR) in congenital and infantile scoliosis. Anterior instrumentation is undertaken when severe curves require an anterior release or when growth arrest procedures are performed. Combined posterior and anterior surgeries are useful in large deformity correction as well as in the prevention of crankshaft phenomenon in skeletally immature individuals. Recently, there is increased interest in the use of minimally invasive fusion for single curves, as well as the use of memory staples or tethers to perform non-fusion scoliosis surgeries.

Scoliosis is a three-dimensional deformity of the spine where the lateral curvature may be combined with vertebral rotation. The current worldwide prevalence is estimated to range from 1-3 % [1, 2]. It is defined by a curvature of at least 10 degrees as measured using the Cobb technique and vertebral rotation on a standing anterior posterior x-ray film combined with the presence of asymmetry on the forward bending test. Scoliosis can be broadly classified into etiology and age at diagnosis.

The categories commonly used to classify scoliosis include

1) Idiopathic (Early and Late Onset)
2) Neuromuscular
3) Congenital and
4) Syndromic

While most cases of scoliosis fall into the idiopathic category, a comprehensive evaluation needs to be performed to rule out an identifiable cause before confirming the diagnosis of idiopathic scoliosis.

Causes

In idiopathic scoliosis, there is no identifiable cause. Recent research points toward patients having a positive family history, central nervous system (CNS) dysfunction in the vestibular system and CNS asymmetry. Collagen, muscle and platelet defects, growth factors, and biomechanical factors are thought to contribute to the cause of idiopathic scoliosis.

A recent study in Asians looked at the levels of bone specific alkaline phosphatase and urine deoxypyridinoline [3]. This study in patients with adolescent idiopathic scoliosis (AIS) aimed at finding a link between bone mass and bone turnover with patients. A strong inverse correlation was found between bone-specific ALP and bone mass in females with AIS. A further conclusion was that bone formation seemed to be stimulated in AIS patients, despite low bone mass density. The bone resorption remained unmodified until 15 years of age. A recent study on leptin hypothesized that circulating serum leptin could result in asymmetrical spine growth during periods of increased upregulation as a result of the sympathetic nervous system or as part of the hypothalamic-pituitary-growth hormone axis [4]. Low melanin has also been implicated as a possible cause in the development of AIS but no conclusive results have been observed in humans [5].

A recent study in the Caucasian population looked at genetic markers of curve progression using a buccal smear based Polymerase Chain Reaction (PCR) analysis. There was good correlation with certain genes for curve progression and further studies will be likely be launched to look at other ethnicities [6].

While there are many hypotheses on growth dysfunction of the developing spine, there has been no definite identifiable etiological factor directly involved in the generation of idiopathic scoliosis.

Neuromuscular scoliosis is associated with neuropathic disorders and myopathic disorders. As defined by the Scoliosis Research Society (SRS), Neuropathic disorders can be broadly classified into upper motor neuron lesions such as cerebral palsy or syringomyelia and lower motor neuron lesions such as spinal muscular atrophy, spinal dysraphism and poliomyelitis. Myopathic disorders include muscular dystrophy and arthrogryposis multiplex congenita. The main etiological factor in such instances involves the muscle imbalance and the effect of gravity on the developing spine. Abnormal pressure at the growth plates results in inhibition of growth. The disproportionate growth in the spine then leads to progressive scoliosis [7]. This theory however has its shortcomings as scoliosis is observed both in flaccid as well as spastic conditions and neither pattern of weakness correlates with a pattern of scoliosis.

The homeobox genes of the HOX class are thought to be responsible in the development of congenital scoliosis [8]. The uncoordinated turning on and off of these genes during weeks 4 to 6 in the embryonic period leads to defects in segmentation and defects of formation of the vertebral bodies. Segmentation disorders of block vertebrate, unilateral bars, and hemivertebra cause a rapidly progressive spinal deformity that can only be halted with surgical intervention. Similarly, formation disorders of wedge vertebra and hemivertebra also result in a child having a rapidly progressive deformity.

Disorders within the spinal cord such as a syrinx or a tethered cord may also produce progressive deformity though the deformity in these conditions may not be as severe initially and the speed of progression of deformity may be slower.

Syndromic scoliosis represents a basket of associations with several clinical conditions such as neurofibromatosis and Marfan's syndrome. Some possible causes in neurofibromatosis include osteomalacia, localized tumour infiltrating bone, endocrine disturbances and mesodermal dysplasia [9].In Marfan's syndrome, a hypothesized underlying cause is the laxity of connective tissue but to date, there has been no conclusive proof.

Symptoms

Most patients with scoliosis are completely asymptomatic. The incidence of back pain in patients with scoliosis in the early stage is equal to that of normal adolescents in the same age. With increasing age and duration of follow up, Weinstein et al. showed that there was an increased incidence of chronic back pain in patients who had scoliosis [10, 11].

As the deformity worsens, the patient may start to experience pain or respiratory symptoms. Pain can be due to the impingement of the ribs onto the pelvic obliquity or can be neuropathic pain from nerve root impingement. Some have also postulated facet joint osteoarthritic pain [11] as a cause of the back pain.

Respiratory symptoms are a result of restrictive lung disease. This can occur in the presence of a large thoracic curve with hypokyphosis [12]. These symptoms are rare as most patients undergo intervention before severe scoliosis of 90-100 degrees (as measured by the Cobb method) is encountered.

Treatment

Each type of scoliosis entails a different type of treatment. While a large proportion of scoliosis can be treated with non-surgical means, surgery may sometimes be required to halt curve progression as well as to restore coronal and sagittal balance.

In the management of scoliosis, all patients with scoliosis will require serial radiographs to document the Cobb angle. Radiographs are also used in pre and post operative assessment. Scoliosis films currently already utilize a lower dose of xray as compared to specific anatomical region xrays. Despite this, patients with scoliosis will potentially be exposed to levels of radiation much higher than the general population. This may in turn put them at a higher risk of carcinogenicity. A recent advance in radiology with a slot scanning radiological device has come to address this problem [13]. The slot scanning device (**EOS** imaging SA., Paris, France) has recently been showed to have superior image quality and clarity of key anatomical landmarks in the radiograph. This comes at an added advantage of lowered radiation dose for the patient.

The aims of surgical management in neuromuscular scoliosis are to treat progression and to address diminished seating ability. In the early stage, bracing with a rigid thoracolumbar spine orthoses (TLSO) is useful in slowing the progression of disease. This is particularly useful in the juvenile years. However, the adolescent growth spurt often is poorly controlled with bracing and will require surgical intervention [14]. Surgical management in neuromuscular scoliosis often involves fusion at an earlier age. Combined anterior and posterior approaches may be used for large curve correction or may be required for patients who have absent posterior elements e.g. myelodysplasia [15]. Intraoperative somatosensory evoked potentials (SSEP) monitoring to detect neural damage has not been useful when performing deformity correction as a standalone tool. Often there is a need to combine with motor evoked potentials as well [16] as this offers better accuracy.

The use of intraoperative halo-femoral traction has also been discussed to allow better correction of deformity. In neuromuscular scoliosis, fixation with rods down to the pelvis (with the Luque-Galverston technique) or the use of iliac screws greatly enhances sitting stability and corrects pelvic obliquity.

Recently, more centers have started to use pedicle screws to achieve fixation across all 3 columns thus enhancing curve correction and providing more secure fixation than sublaminar wires.

Intraoperatively, the use of Halo-femoral traction as well as temporary internal distraction has been used to successfully perform correction without the need for an anterior procedure.

The aim of surgery is a return to the preoperative functional level with a solidly fused spine in coronal and sagittal plane balance over a level pelvis.

In situations where severe deformity exists, vertebral column resection (VCR) or osteotomies from the posterior approach has been used. While this entails a longer operating time and larger blood loss, it has been shown to be a powerful tool in correcting large deformities and restoring pelvic balance [17].

The treatment of congenital scoliosis is challenging. Unilateral unsegmented bars with or without contralateral hemivertebra cause the most rapid progression. Up to 30 percent of such cases may have intraspinal pathology. At the initial presentation, patients may require a magnetic resonance imaging (MRI) of the spine if they present with a large deformity. Rapid curve progression is another indication for a MRI scan. The reason for this is to ensure that Chiari malformations or intraspinal pathology such as tumours or a syrinx is excluded as a cause of the rapid deformity.

The options for treatment in congenital scoliosis include posterior fusion with or without instrumentation, combined anterior and posterior fusion, growth arrest procedures, hemivertebra excision, vertebrectomy, the use of the vertical expandable prosthetic titanium rib (VEPTR) and the use of growing rods.

In-situ posterior fusion is often performed for small curvatures that are anticipated to worsen. This should not be undertaken without consideration to the risk of crankshaft phenomenon (bending of the fused segment) which occurs when there is significant anterior growth left [18]. In such instances, combined anterior and posterior fusion should be considered.

The use of the VEPTR was initially targeted at treatment of thoracic insufficiency syndrome, aiming to allow the child to have adequate maturation of the lung [19]. Since its introduction, its use has slowly expanded to include early onset scoliosis. Finally, the use of growing rods with a pedicle screw caudal construct has been used as well [20]. These non-fusion instrumented surgeries have an aim of allowing maximal spine growth and act as a guiding axis to prevent deformity. They will require eventual removal of implants and fusion when the child reaches skeletal maturity.

When considering the spectrum of idiopathic scoliosis, early onset scoliosis is differentiated from late onset scoliosis as each entity is treated differently. The definition of early onset scoliosis (EOS) is based on the greatest amount of growth in the thoracic cavity and spine during the ages of 0-5.

Early Onset Scoliosis

The treatment of EOS can be broadly classified into non-surgical and surgical. Non-surgical treatment encompasses observation when the Cobb angle is less than 25 degrees and when the rib vertebral angle difference (RVAD) is less than 20 degrees. Should there be documented progression or if at first presentation, the child already has a curve of 35 degrees, orthotic treatment is indicated. Orthotic treatment encompasses casting under general anaesthesia with 6 weekly changes to obtain maximal correction prior to using a cervicothoracolumbar orthosis (CTLSO) for maintainence of correction and prevention of further progression [21]. Orthotic use is continued for 2 years until the Cobb angle and the RVAD is stable.

Surgical treatment for EOS is targeted at individuals who fail orthotic treatment and demonstrate curve progression. Those with Cobb angles of more than 45 degrees or demonstrate thoracic insufficiency syndrome are also candidates for surgical treatment.

Surgical treatment in a young patient often entails non-fusion spinal instrumentation. Growing rods have showed reasonable outcomes in preventing deformity and at the same time allowing continued growth in the thoracolumbar spine [20]. Another modality of interest is the use of VEPTR in patients with EOS and thoracic insufficiency syndrome [19]. While these devices have been effective in controlling deformity, they are all associated with a higher than normal complication rate. Complications include implant related complications such as hook loosening, rod breakage, skin prominence, and scarring as a result of repeated lengthening procedures that are continually performed as the child grows.

Late Onset Scoliosis (LOS)

LOS encompasses juvenile idiopathic scoliosis and adolescent idiopathic scoliosis. Left sided thoracic curves, atypical curve shapes, rapid progression, male gender, and abnormal abdominal reflexes are factors associated with coexistant neural axis deformity (e.g. syrinx). These patients will often require an MRI scan of the entire spine to be performed [22].

Juvenile scoliosis can be braced when within the 25 to 50 degree range and non-fusion spine instrumentation surgery is indicated when the curve exceeds 50 to 60 degrees. Current treatment modalities include dual growing rod constructs [20] with caudal and cephalad pedicle screw anchors, or with the use of rib hooks as a form of hybrid fixation. These represent modifications to the original use of Harrington rods in a non-fusion surgery. The use of staples as a form of hemiepiphysiodesis has also been described [23]. More recently, thoracoscopically inserted anterior tethering devices have generated interest as a minimally invasive way in achieving fusionless surgery. Long term studies are currently still not available at this stage but early results have proved promising [24].

The vast majority of LOS cases are adolescent idiopathic scoliosis (AIS). AIS also represents the commonest type of scoliosis seen worldwide. The treatment of AIS is dependent on the magnitude of the curve and the maturity of the spine. When the Cobb angle is less than 20 degrees and the RVAD is less than 20 degrees, the patient is observed with 6 monthly or once yearly full length xray films. Curve progression beyond 25 degrees is best treated with a thoracolumbar brace if the spine is skeletally immature. A combination of menstrual history, Tanner staging, and radiological features of the risser stage are used to determine the skeletal maturity of the spine. Risser stage 0-2 curves are amenable to bracing. Bracing involves the use of dynamic or rigid thoracolumbar orthoses, and the brace should be worn for more than 20 hours a day to prevent progression. Common types of braces available are dynamic bracing such as the SpineCor® brace, or rigid bracing such as the Boston thoracolumbar orthoses [25, 26]. While these braces have showed effective outcome in the management of scoliosis, compliance to the usage of the brace for the prescribed daily duration forms the greatest challenge facing the treating orthopaedists, parents and children. This is particularly true for children residing in tropical countries where heat and humidity form deterrence in wearing the brace for such extended lengths of time.

In patients who are skeletally mature, but who continue to show progression in their Cobb angles, they can be counseled for deformity correction and fusion. The Lenke classification has been used with success in determining the extent of fusion required based on the rigidity of the curve [27].

Weinstein et al. showed previously that patients who have curves of more than 50 degrees would have a high risk of having curve progression of 0.5 to 1 degree per year following skeletal maturity [28]. Wong et al. also showed similar results in the Asian context [29].

Surgical management of the thoracolumbar curve involves posterior, anterior or combined anterior and posterior instrumentation and fusion. Curve flexibility as demonstrated on the bending films have showed to be useful in predicting the correctability of such curves.

In order to achieve maximal correction of the deformity, several advances in implant technology as well as biologics in enhancing early spine fusion have emerged in the last 10 years. The use of the pedicle screw has impacted the practice of spine surgery as increasing number of authors have reported better correction and maintenance of correction with the aid of all pedicle screw constructs [30]. Monoaxial screws at the curve apex have also showed better curve control and rotation as compared to polyaxial screws [31]. The use of cobalt chrome rods as compared to titanium rods as a stiffer and more rigid guide to deformity correction has also impacted the operative choices in scoliosis management.

With the advent of minimally invasive spine surgery in treating adult deformity, recent advances have been made in performing minimally invasive surgery for adolescent scoliosis.

Video assisted thoracoscopic surgery (VATS) with intervertebral disc releases and fusion in Lenke 1 curves has been used successfully. Though these surgeries have a longer operating time, they showed distinct improvements in reducing blood requirements as well as improved cosmesis [32]. Recent data has showed that posterior only fixation has had equal success in achieving correction in thoracolumbar scoliosis [33].

Most recently, many centers have started using posterior minimally invasive surgery (MIS) for AIS. The limitations of such surgery include curve length and may be limited at present to single curves [34]. It remains to be seen if long term outcomes will be as effective as traditional posterior open surgery. Interestingly, due to the reduced surface for application of bone graft, bone morphogenic proteins (BMP) has been used to achieve fusion in posterior MIS surgery for scoliosis [35]. However, caution should be taken against the use of high dosages due to recent concerns on carcinogenicity and osteolysis [36].

Post surgery, patients are excluded from strenuous exercise and contact sports for up to a year while awaiting fusion. Once fusion is successful, they may engage in routine sporting activity and can be allowed gradual return to contact sports [37].

Conclusion

Scoliosis remains a challenging condition to manage, particularly in the immature individual. While advances have been made with regards to the predictability of curve progression, there are still few answers that point to a direct cause of scoliosis which can be treated successfully. Compliance to orthotic treatment remains the mainstay of therapy and operative intervention is often required to prevent curve progression and maintain balance. In time, continued innovation and design will change the surgical approach in managing scoliosis and the future looks toward anterior and posterior forms of minimally invasive surgery in taking on the challenges of managing this condition.

References

[1] Lonstein JE. Screening for spinal deformities in Minnesota schools. *Clin Orthop* 1977;126:33–42.

[2] Ohtsuka Y, Yamagata M, Arai S, et al. School screening for scoliosis by the Chiba University Medical School screening program. *Spine* 1988;13:1251–7.

[3] C.S.K. Cheung, W.T.K. Lee, Y.K. Tse, K.M. Lee, X. Guo, L. Qin, et al., Generalized osteopenia in adolescent idiopathic scoliosis—association with abnormal pubertal growth,bone turnover, and calcium intake? *Spine* 31 (3) (2006) 330–338.

[4] R.G. Burwell, R.K. Auljia, M.P. Grevitt, P.H. Dangerfield, A. Moulton, T.L. Randell,et al., Pathogenesis of adolescent idiopathic scoliosis in girls—a double neuro-osseous theory involving disharmony between two nervous systems, somatic and autonomic expressed in the spine and trunk: possible dependency on sympathetic nervous system and hormones with implications for medical therapy, *Scoliosis* 4 (2009) 24.

[5] M. Machida, J. Dubousset, T. Yamada, J. Kimura, Serum melatonin levels in adolescent idiopathic scoliosis prediction and prevention for curve progression—a prospective study,*J. Pineal Res.* 46 (3) (2009) 344–348.

[6] Ward K, Ogilvie JW, Singleton MV, Chettier R, Engler G, Nelson LM. Validation of DNA-based prognostic testing to predict spinal curve

progression in adolescent idiopathic scoliosis. *Spine* (Phila Pa 1976). 2010 Dec 1;35(25):E1455-64.

[7] Newton PO, Faro F, Wenger D, et al. Neuromuscular Scoliosis. In HerkowitzHN, Garfin SR, Eismont FJ, Bell GR, Balderston RA, Editors. Rothman and Simeone The Spine 5th Ed. Philadelphia Saunders:2006 p535-64.

[8] Miller NH, Marosy B, Justice CM, Novak SM, Tang EY, Boyce P, Pettengil J, Doheny KF, Pugh EW, Wilson AF.Linkage analysis of genetic loci for kyphoscoliosis on chromosomes 5p13, 13q13.3, and 13q32. *Am J Med Genet* A. 2006 May 15;140(10):1059-68.

[9] Crawford AH, Herrera-Soto J. Orthop Clin North Am. 2007 Oct;38(4):553-62, vii. Scoliosis associated with neurofibromatosis.

[10] Weinstein SL, Zavala DC, Ponseti IV. Idiopathic scoliosis: Long-term follow-up and prognosis in untreated patients. *J Bone Joint Surg* [Am] 1981;63:702–12.

[11] Weinstein SL, Dolan LA, Spratt KF, Peterson K, Spoonamore, M: Natural History of Adolescent Idiopathic Scoliosis: Back Pain at 50 years. Presented at the annual meeting of the Scoliosis Research Society, September, 1998; New York, NY.

[12] Winter RB, Lovell WW, Moe JH. Excessive thoracic lordosis and loss of pulmonary function in patients with idiopathic scoliosis. *J Bone Joint Surg* [Am] 1975;57:972–7.

[13] Deschênes S, Charron G, Beaudoin G, Labelle H, Dubois J, Miron MC, Parent S. Diagnostic imaging of spinal deformities: reducing patients radiation dose with a new slot-scanning X-ray imager. *Spine* (Phila Pa 1976). 2010 Apr 20;35(9):989-94.

[14] Sussman MD, Little D, Alley RM, McCoig JA. Posterior instrumentation and fusion of the thoracolumbar spine for treatment of neuromuscular scoliosis. *J Pediatr Orthop*. May-Jun 1996;16(3):304-13.

[15] Sarwahi V, Sarwark JF, Schafer MF, et al. Standards in anterior spine surgery in pediatric patients with neuromuscular scoliosis. *J Pediatr Orthop*. Nov-Dec 2001;21(6):756-60.

[16] Owen, J H; Sponseller, P D; Szymanski, J; Hurdle, M. Efficacy of multimodality spinal cord monitoring during surgery for neuromuscular scoliosis. *Spine* 20 (13): 1480-8, 1995 Jul 1.

[17] Sponseller PD, Jain A, Lenke LG, Shah SA, Sucato DJ, Emans JB, Newton PO. Vertebral Column Resection in Children with Neuromuscular Spine Deformity. *Spine* (Phila Pa 1976). 2011 Dec 13.

[18] Kesling KL, Lonstein JE, Denis F, Perra JH, Schwender JD, Transfeldt EE, et al. The crankshaft phenomenon after posterior spinal arthrodesis for congenital scoliosis: a review of 54 patients. *Spine*. Feb 1 2003;28(3):267-71.
[19] Motoyama EK, Deeney VF, Fine GF, et al. Effects on lung function of multiple expansion thoracoplasty in children with thoracic insufficiency syndrome: a longitudinal study. *Spine*. 2006;31(3):284-90.
[20] Akbarnia BA., Marks DS, Boachie-Adjei O, et al. Dual growing rod technique for the treatment of progressive early-onset scoliosis: a multicenter study. *Spine*. 2005;30(17 Suppl):S46-57.
[21] D'Astous JL, Sanders JO. Casting and traction treatment methods for scoliosis. *Orthop Clin North Am*. Oct 2007;38(4):477-84
[22] Nakahara D, Yonezawa I, Kobanawa K, Sakoda J, Nojiri H, Kamano S, Okuda T, Kurosawa H. Magnetic resonance imaging evaluation of patients with idiopathic scoliosis: a prospective study of four hundred seventy-two outpatients. *Spine* (Phila Pa 1976). 2011 Apr 1;36(7):E482-5.
[23] O'leary PT, Sturm PF, Hammerberg KW, Lubicky JP, Mardjetko SM. Convex hemiepiphysiodesis: the limits of vertebral stapling. *Spine* (Phila Pa 1976). 2011 Sep 1;36(19):1579-83.
[24] Newton PO, Farnsworth CL, Upasani VV, Chambers RC, Varley E, Tsutsui S. Effects of intraoperative tensioning of an anterolateral spinal tether on spinal growth modulation in a porcine model. *Spine* (Phila Pa 1976). 2011 Jan 15;36(2):109-17.
[25] Coillard C, Vachon V, Circo AB, Beauséjour M, Rivard CH. Effectiveness of the SpineCor brace based on the new standardized criteria proposed by the scoliosis research society for adolescent idiopathic scoliosis. *J Pediatr Orthop*. 2007 Jun;27(4):375-9.
[26] Wiley JW, Thomson JD, Mitchell TM, Smith BG, Banta JV. Effectiveness of the boston brace in treatment of large curves in adolescent idiopathic scoliosis. *Spine* (Phila Pa 1976). 2000 Sep 15;25(18):2326-32.
[27] Lenke LG, Betz RR, Harms J, Bridwell KH, Clements DH, Lowe TG, Blanke K.J Adolescent idiopathic scoliosis: a new classification to determine extent of spinal arthrodesis. *Bone Joint Surg Am*. 2001 Aug;83-A(8):1169-81.
[28] Weinstein SL.Natural history *Spine* (Phila Pa 1976). 1999 Dec 15;24(24):2592-600. Review.

[29] Tan KJ, Moe MM, Vaithinathan R, Wong HK. Curve progression in idiopathic scoliosis: follow-up study to skeletal maturity. *Spine* (Phila Pa 1976). 2009 Apr 1;34(7):697-700.
[30] Cuartas E, Rasouli A, O'Brien M, Shufflebarger HL. Use of all-pedicle-screw constructs in the treatment of adolescent idiopathic scoliosis. *J Am Acad Orthop Surg.* 2009 Sep;17(9):550-61.
[31] Lonner BS, Auerbach JD, Boachie-Adjei O, Shah SA, Hosogane N, Newton PO.Treatment of thoracic scoliosis *Spine* (Phila Pa 1976). 2009 Apr 15;34(8):845-51
[32] Wong HK, Hee HT, Yu Z, Wong D. Results of thoracoscopic instrumented fusion versus conventional posterior instrumented fusion in adolescent idiopathic scoliosis undergoing selective thoracic fusion. *Spine* (Phila Pa 1976). 2004 Sep 15;29(18):2031-8
[33] Hee HT, Yu ZR, Wong HK Comparison of segmental pedicle screw instrumentation versus anterior instrumentation in adolescent idiopathic Spine (Phila Pa 1976). 2007 Jun 15;32(14):1533-42.
[34] Sarwahi V, Wollowick AL, Sugarman EP, Horn JJ, Gambassi M, Amaral TD. Minimally invasive scoliosis surgery: an innovative technique in patients with adolescent idiopathic scoliosis. *Scoliosis.* 2011 Aug 11;6:16.
[35] Betz RR, Lavelle WF, Samdani AF. Bone grafting options in children. *Spine* (Phila Pa 1976) 2010;35:1648–1654
[36] Carragee EJ, Hurwitz EL, Weiner BK. A critical review of recombinant human *Spine J.* 2011 Jun;11(6):471-91. Review.
[37] Rubery PT, Bradford DS. Athletic activity after spine Spine (Phila Pa 1976). 2002 Feb 15;27(4):423-

In: Scoliosis: Causes, Symptoms and Treatment   ISBN: 978-1-62081-007-1
Editors: A. Bessette et al.   © 2012 Nova Science Publishers, Inc.

Chapter V

A New Physical Therapy Intervention for Scoliosis

Clare Lewis
Department of Physical Therapy,
California State University, Sacramento, CA, US

Abstract

Introduction: Various non-invasive treatments have been used as interventions for mild to moderate scoliosis, those that are not severe enough to require surgery (40 degrees or less). While many of these have not shown to be efficacious, others have documented indicators of improvement. Despite the improvements obtained with conservative methods, individuals with scoliosis would benefit from more effective therapies. Purpose: To further study the effectiveness of the ATM2™ for treatment of scoliosis. The ATM2™ was previously shown to improve a scoliotic curve, in a published case study. Methods: Thirty-eight subjects were put on a therapy intervention using the ATM2™ for eight to twenty sessions. Results: All subjects saw improvements in a variety of variables. Discussion: The ATM2™ has shown to be a viable non-invasive intervention for the treatment of mild to moderate scoliosis.

Introduction

This chapter will review traditional non-invasive interventions for scoliosis. It will discuss the efficacy or lack of efficacy for electrical stimulation, bracing, traditional exercises, manipulation and vestibular rehabilitation. This chapter will introduce the ATM2™ as a new physical therapy intervention for scoliosis and discuss published research results thus far.

A Brief Definitoin of Scoliosis

Scoliosis is used to describe an abnormal curvature of the spine, but it is not in itself a disease or a diagnosis. The curvature of the spine from scoliosis is from side to side and may develop as a single curve (shaped like the letter C) or as two curves (shaped like the letter S).

Scoliosis usually develops in the upper back (thoracic spine) or area between the upper back and lower back (the thoracolumbar area of the spine). It may also occur just in the lower back (lumbar spine). Scoliosis can be caused by congenital, developmental or degenerative problems, but most cases of scoliosis actually have no known cause [1,2] (although very recently a gene marker has been found for scoliosis [3]) and this is known as idiopathic scoliosis. While there are many forms of scoliosis, four of the most common ones include:

- Congenital scoliosis
- Neuromuscular scoliosis
- Degenerative scoliosis
- Idiopathic scoliosis

Because it most often occurs during adolescence, idiopathic scoliosis is sometimes called *adolescent scoliosis*. Scoliosis does not come from activities such as sports involvement, wearing a backpack, sleeping positions, posture, or minor leg length differences. [1,2]

Idiopathic Scoliosis

This is by far the most prevalent form of scoliosis and occurs to some degree in approximately one half million adolescents in the US. Scoliosis has been seen to occur in families and thus the search for a genetic link (noted above).

Idiopathic scoliosis is usually categorized into three age groups:

- From birth to 3 years old - called *infantile scoliosis*.
- From 3 to 9 years old - called *juvenile scoliosis*.
- From 10 to 18 years old – called *adolescent scoliosis*.

This last category of scoliosis, which occurs from 10 to 18 years old, comprises approximately 80 percent of all cases of idiopathic scoliosis.

The risk of curvature progression is increased during puberty, when the growth rate of the body is the fastest. Scoliosis with significant curvature of the spine is much more prevalent in girls than in boys, and girls are eight times more likely to need treatment for scoliosis, because they tend to have curves that are much more likely to progress. Still, the majority of all cases of scoliosis are mild and do not require treatment.

It is important to note that although idiopathic scoliosis results in spinal deformity, it is not typically a cause of back pain. Of course, people with scoliosis can develop back pain, just as most of the adult population can develop back pain. However, it has never been found that people with idiopathic scoliosis are any more likely to develop back pain than the rest of the population.

In children and teenagers, scoliosis often does not have any noticeable symptoms, therefore scoliosis is often not noticeable until the curve has progressed significantly.

When viewed from the side, a healthy spine curves inward in the lower back (lordosis) and outward in the upper back. When viewed from the back, a spine with normal curves appears as a straight line down the back. A person with scoliosis, however, will appear to have a side-to-side curve in their spine because of a lateral, or sideways, curvature of the spine.

There are several common physical signs that may indicate scoliosis. As noted above, any type of back pain is not usually considered a scoliosis symptom. Most typically, signs of scoliosis may include one or several of the following:

- One shoulder is higher than the other
- One shoulder blade sticks out more than the other
- One side of the rib cage appears higher than the other
- One hip appears higher or more prominent than the other
- The waist appears uneven
- The body tilts to one side
- One leg may appear shorter than the other

Frequently, a scoliosis curve in the spine is first diagnosed in school exams or in a regular check up with a pediatrician. Most students are given the *Adam's forward bend* test routinely in school when they are in fifth and/or sixth grade to determine whether or not they may have scoliosis. The test involves the student bending forward with arms stretched downward toward the floor and knees straight, while being observed from behind by a healthcare professional. This angle most clearly shows any asymmetry in the spine and/or trunk of the adolescent's body.

Because a scoliosis curvature is usually in the thoracic or thoracolumbar spine (upper back or mid back), if a rib hump or asymmetry of the lumbar spine is found, or if the shoulders are different heights, it is possible that the individual has scoliosis. An x-ray is ordered to both confirm the scoliosis diagnosis and check on the magnitude of the spinal curvature. The x-ray will also give some indication as to the skeletal maturity of the patient, which may influence treatment decisions.

In rare instances a physician may also request an MRI scan of the thoracic and/or cervical. If there are any neurological deficits that would indicate impingement of the spinal cord (e.g. brisk reflex), if there is a left-sided thoracic curvature (they are almost always right sided), or if the child is very young (8 to 11 years old), an MRI scan is advisable to examine the possibility of an intra-canal spinal lesion, which can cause scoliosis.

Depending on the results of the physician's clinical evaluation and the diagnostic tests, a scoliosis treatment plan will be recommended that may include observation, bracing, exercise and possibly surgery to reduce or correct the spinal curve.

Decision for scoliosis treatment decisions are primarily based on two factors:

- The *skeletal maturity of the patient* (or rather, how much more growth can be expected)

- The *degree of spinal curvature*.

The way scoliosis curves behave is fairly well understood. Basically, the younger the patient and the bigger the curve, the more likely the curve is to progress, therefore early detection is essential for scoliosis treatment to be most effective.

The scoliosis curvature is measured on x-rays by what is known as the Cobb method, and this form of measurement is accurate to within 3 to 5 degrees.

Curves that are less than 10 degrees are not considered to even represent scoliosis but rather just spinal asymmetry. These types of curves are extremely unlikely to progress and generally do not need any treatment. If the child is very young and physically immature, then the progress of the curve can be followed during the child's regular check up with his or her pediatrician. If the curve is noticed to progress beyond 20 degrees, then the child should be referred to an orthopedic surgeon with expertise in scoliosis for continued treatment.

As mentioned earlier, pain is not a typical symptom of scoliosis. Back pain in a child or teen that has scoliosis may indicate another problem, and a pediatrician and/or spine specialist should evaluate the child. If a child or teen has back pain and also has scoliosis, it is very important that he or she see a doctor to find out the cause of the pain, as it is probably something other than the scoliosis causing the back pain and may require treatment. Neurologic injury is also a very rare presenting symptom of scoliosis. [1,2]

The Need for Effective Treatment for Scoliosis

Scoliosis affects approximately 2% of the population. As a result of the changing appearance of the back from the abnormal spinal curvature, the self-esteem of a person who has scoliosis can be dramatically affected. If scoliosis is allowed to progress, pain can become an eventual symptom and pain levels can result in secondary impairments, which if left untreated, can become severe. [4]

For curves that do no require surgery, many different physical therapy treatments have been utilized to treat scoliosis including electrical muscle stimulation, bracing, various exercise programs, and manipulation among others. Unfortunately these have not been found to be very effective treatments for scoliosis.

The ATM2™, is a vertical treatment table, that was developed by a physical therapist trained in "Mulligan Techniques," also know as Mobilization with Movement (MWM). MWM was developed by Brian Mulligan, a physiotherapist in New Zealand. The difference between classic mobilization and MWM is that the joint being mobilized is being actively moved at the same time as a mobilizing force is applied. Clinical evidence has been documented for the efficacy of the ATM2™ when used with patients who have LBP, hip problems, shoulder problems and cervical problems. The ATM2™ was also found to be effective in helping to reverse the curves in a patient with scoliosis who was actually being treated for a frozen shoulder in a recently published case study. [5] Further study has been conducted to determine if the ATM2™ could be an effective physical therapy modality to specifically treat scoliosis by reversing the curves of subjects with scoliosis. The results of ongoing study have been quite promising that the ATM2™ is effective in not only helping to decrease pain and increase range of motion (ROM) but also significantly improve the posture and appearance of the spine in one who has scoliosis.

Electrical Stimulation for Scoliosis

The usual protocol for using electrical stimulation to treat scoliosis is to place the electrodes so that they are on the convex side(s) of the spinal curve. The convex side of the curve is considered to be the long and weak side, while the concave side of the curve is considered to be strong and tight. The intention of the treatment is to stimulate those long and weak muscles and thereby result in the ability of the newly strong muscles to pull the spine into a more vertical position.

Clinical studies have not shown efficacy for electrical stimulation as a treatment intervention for scoliosis. [6,7]

Bracing

Bracing is designed to stop the progression of the spinal curve, but it does not reduce the amount of angulation already present. The majority of curve progression happens during a child's growth phase, and once the growth has ended, there is little likelihood of progression of a curve. Therefore, bracing is continued until the child is skeletally mature and finished growing. Unfortunately, even with appropriate bracing, some scoliosis spinal curves will continue to progress. For these cases, especially if the child is very young, bracing may still be continued to allow the child to grow before fusing the spine. [1]

Scoliosis Exercise for Pain Relief and Curve Correction

Traditional physical therapy exercises for scoliosis consist of moves that are designed to help stretch out the concave side of the curve and to strengthen the convex side of the curve. These are often done on the floor on a mat starting from a quadruped or side lying position. Hanging from a bar is also included in these exercises. [8] In one extensive review of the literature, authors concluded that the effectiveness of exercise is not yet established, but might be promising. [8]

Manipulation

A search of the literature finds variable results about the effectiveness of manipulation for scoliosis. For example, according to Dr. Lantz, "Full-spine chiropractic adjustments with heel lifts and lifestyle counseling are not effective in reducing the severity of scoliotic curves." [9]

Dr. Mark Morningstar on the other hand had a different viewpoint when he wrote that scoliosis treatment using a combination of manipulative and rehabilitative therapy was effective. His results revealed after 4-6 weeks of treatment, that the entire sample size studied averaged a 62% reduction in their Cobb angle measurements. [10]

Dennis Woggon, BSc, DC states, "Spinal Manipulation Therapy and Chiropractic Adjustments both may have a detrimental effect on Scoliosis by mobilizing compensated fixated stabilizing spinal units and that both of these interventions may actually increase scoliosis." He summarizes that symptomatic care is preferable and is the method taught in most Chiropractic Colleges. [11]

Scroth Method

The Schroth Method incorporates a three dimensional therapy to reshape the ribcage and reduce the deformity associated with Scoliosis. The aim of these scoliosis specific exercises for adults and children should reduce the incidence of scoliosis progression, reduce postural rotation, improve mobility, improve postural stability, reduce pain, and improve cardiopulmonary function. In a study of 813 patients who completed the Schroth in-patient program, results showed an increase in chest expansion of more that 20%. The conclusion of the study author was that a course of inpatient treatment of the Schroth method resulted in an increase in vital capacity and chest expansion. [6] In another study by Weis, 118 inpatients with an average Cobb measurement of 31 degrees were treated with the Schroth method and tracked for four years. 16.1% had progression of their curve, 68.7% had stabilization of their curve and 15.2% had an improvement of more than 5 degrees. The author concluded that in patients with idiopathic scoliosis, the Schroth method appeared to retard the natural progression of scoliosis compared to the natural history of scoliosis without intervention. [12]

Vestibular Rehabilitation

Vestibular disturbances have been reported in scoliosis patients. [13,14] In one study, it was found that children with a slight imbalance in the activity of vestibular complex was responsible for the spinal curvature which characterizes Idiopathic Scoliosis. [14]

It has been reported that vestibular dysfunction left untreated influences postural tone, in particular extensor musculature activity during dynamic balance. Studies confirm abnormal activation of extensor musculature during walking in scoliosis patients. [15] Jensen et al recommend that a neurological examination, including assessment of vestibular function, be incorporated into screening methods for scoliosis. [16]

Vestibular training has been used to optimize postural muscle synergies through repetitive movement therapy and vestibular rehabilitation. A study in Spine reported that significant differences were found between patients with right convex curves and those with left convex curves in the distribution of eye predominance and in labyrinthine sensitivity. [17]

Another interesting finding that has been reported in the literature is the adolescent population with vestibular pathology are often without symptoms, much in the same way they are typically without pain. On the other hand, the adult population often suffers from dizziness, imbalance, anxiety and vestibular headaches as a direct result of their vestibular disorder, and experience chronic pain syndromes as well. To date, vestibular rehabilitation and, really, any rehabilitation of movement remains controversial in the United States. [18]

The ATM2™ in the Treatment of Scoliosis

The ATM2™ was never intended as a treatment specifically for treating scoliosis so it was with much surprise when it was discovered by accident, that a patient who was being treated for a frozen shoulder was also getting as a secondary benefit an improvement of her longstanding scoliosis and kyphosis. After her first treatment, the patient explained, that she immediately noticed when she sat in her car that her head was touching the headrest of her car seat. She had never been able to do this before because her thoracic kyphosis prevented her head from going back far enough to touch the headrest. At her second treatment session documentation of the patients posture began along with other measurements related to her scoliosis. After several treatment sessions aimed at treating her postural faults, significant improvements were evident in the patient's posture from the ATM2™ interventions alone. This was the first time such documentation had taken place for postural improvements noted while using the ATM2™, although many clinicians have noted similar improvements in their patients' posture after treatment with the ATM2™.[5]

Since publication of the above case study, further study was undertaken to determine if the ATM2™ would be effective in treating scoliosis by reversing the curves of other subjects with mild to moderate scoliosis.

The following information is from the current study:

Metods and Materials

38 subjects (34 female, 4 male) with a diagnosis of scoliosis were recruited from a scoliosis support group and by advertising to local physicians.

Inclusion criteria were as follows: subjects were between the ages of 12-65 with a diagnosis of scoliosis curve between 20° and 50°. Exclusion criteria were as follows: a previous surgery to correct the curve, current pregnancy, any serious medical co-morbidities, any history of claustrophobia or currently suffering from severe back pain that required medication. Subjects were put on the ATM2™ and performed *pain free* movements in several directions. All subjects performed resisted extension and side bending into their convexity in order to move into the direction that reversed their curve. The subjects were progressed from 1 set of 10 repetitions to 3 sets of 10 repetitions in each direction. All subjects completed at least 1 round of treatments, which consisted of between 8-10 sessions. Some subjects who were available completed a second round of sessions for a total of 20 treatments. Objective measures utilized in this study included:

- Numeric Pain Rating Scale
- SF 36
- Oswestry Disability Index
- Cobb angles from pre and post intervention x-rays
- Height
- Trunk ROM measurements including:
    o Flexion and Extension (measured using double inclinometer method)
    o Side Bending (measured fingertips to floor, with measuring tape)
    o Rotation (measured with goniometer)

Results

All outcome measures were analyzed using a paired t-test. Multiple outcome measures Demonstrated statistically significant change at the 0.05 Level of Significance including:

- Right Side Bending ($p=0.007$)
- Right Rotation ($p=0.003$)
- Left Rotation ($p=3.07 \times 10^{-5}$)
- Trunk Flexion ($p=0.1$) *(most subjects able to touch fingertips to floor at the start of the study before any intervention)
- Height ($p=.005$)

- Numeric Pain Rating (p=0.0002)
- Oswestry Disability Index (p=0.01)

Five subjects were able to obtain pre and post treatment x-rays. Decreases in angle of curvaturewere seen in three subjects when determining Cobb angles. Statistical analysis was not run because of the small sample size. Cobb angles improved or were unchanged for the 5 subjects for whom x-rays were obtained. The Minimal Clinically Significant Difference for Cobb angles is ~7 degrees in adolescents (MCSD not available for adults). SF-36 data showed statistical significance for the majority of variables.

Discussion and Conclusion

This study was done to determine if the ATM2™ can treat scoliosis by reversing spinal curvature. The hypothesis for efficacy is that by stabilizing a scoliotic curve, and then moving into resistance, the apex of the curve would receive mobilization while the active movement from the subject would achieve neuromuscular re-education of the supporting musculature. X-rays taken before and after intervention showed decreases in Cobb angles for three subjects who were able to provide post treatment x-rays. Before and after photos also showed changes in those who began with greater spinal curvatures. Some subjects reported they received comments about improved posture from family and friends. Subjects also reported improved self-image as a result of the study. In addition, several objective measures of ROM, as well as height, pain rating and the Oswestry Disability Index have been found to have statistically significant improvement after treatment with the ATM2™. The ATM2™ was shown to be effective in reducing the Cobb angles of three subjects, as well as showing observable postural changes with pre and post intervention posture pictures. Based on the results of this study, treatment with the ATM2™ positively affects perceived level of health, self-image, visible posture correction, ROM, height, and self-reported disability measures.

Continued study is ongoing with the goal of improving the power of current the study by increasing the sample size, especially with regard to Cobb angle data. The ATM2™ intervention continues to provide significant positive results for the subjects who have been involved in our study. [19]

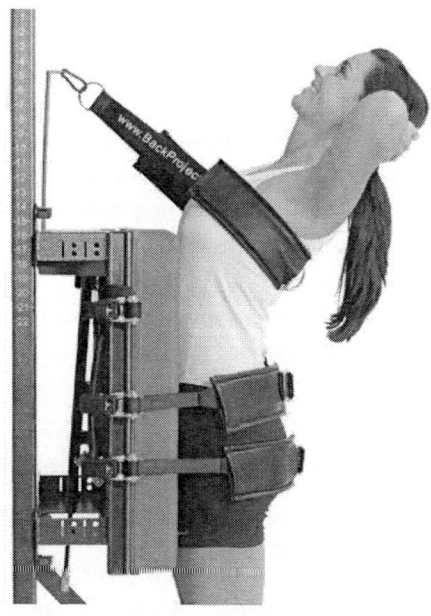

Figure 1. The ATM2™.

References

[1] Mayo clinic authors (2009) http://www.mayoclinic.com/health/scoliosis/DS00194/DSECTION=causes
[2] Diers authors (2011) http://www.diers.de/formetric-en/
[3] Sadit-ali, A (2011) http://www.ncbi.nlm.nih.gov/pubmed/21814337
[4] Scoliosis Research Society authors (2011) http://www.SRS.org/htm/glossary/ medterms.htm
[5] Lewis, C.; Erhard, R.; Drysdale, G. Kyphoscoliosis Improvement While Treating a Patient for Adhesive Capsulitis Using the Active Therapeutic Movement Version 2. JMPT 2008, Vol, 31, pp 715-22.
[6] Lenssinck, M.; et al. Electrical Stimulation Versus Brace in Treatment of Idiopathic Scoliosis Effect of Bracing and Other Conservative Interventions in the Treatment of Idiopathic Scoliosis in Adolescents: A Systematic Review of Clinical Trials. *Phys. Ther,* 2005 Vol 85, no.12 1329-1339.
[7] Durham, J. Moskowitz; A. Whitney, J. Surface Electrical Stimulation Versus Brace in Treatment of Idiopathic Scolisis. *Spine*, 1990 Vol 15, #9 pp. 888-892.

[8] Weiss, R. The Effect of an Exercise Program on Vital Capacity and Rib Mobility in Patients with Idiopathic Scoliosis. *Spine*, 1991 Vol 16, #1 pp 88-93.
[9] Lantz, C.; Chen, J. Effect of chiropractic intervention on small scoliotic curves in younger subjects: A time-series cohort design. *JMPT*, 2001 Vol 6, pp 385-93.
[10] http://www.biomedcentral.com/1471-2474/5/32
[11] http://www.clear-institute.org/Portals/0/docs/ScoliosisCC.pdf
[12] Lehnert-Schroth, C. (2007) The Schroth Three-Dimensional Treatment. Oxford:Elsevier.
[13] Woods, et al. Decreased Incidence of Scoliosis in Hearing-Impaired Children.| Implications for a Neurologic Basis for Idiopathic Scoliosis. *Spine*, 1995 Vol 20, pp.776-80.
[14] Byl, N.; Gray, J. Complex balance reactions in different sensory conditions: Adolescents with and without idiopathic scoliosis. *J. of orthopedic. research*, 2005 Vol 11, pp 215-227.
[15] Manzoni, D; Zeno S. Vestibular Mechanisms Involved in Idiopathic Scoliosis. *Arch. Ital. Biol.* 2002 Vol 140, pp 67-80.
[16] Jensen, G.; Wilson, K. Horizontal Postrotatory Nystagmus Response in Females with Adolescent Idiopathic Scoliosis. *Phys. Ther*, 1979 Vol 59, pp 1226-1233.
[17] Sahlstrand T. Vestibular dysfunction has been linked to abnormal spinal curvatures. Treatment plans. *Spine* 1980 Vol 5 pp 512-8.
[18] Guo, Xia MD et al. Balance Control in Adolescents With Idiopathic Scoliosis and Disturbed Somatosensory Function. *Spine*, 2006 Vol 31, pp 437-40.
[19] Lewis study in progress.

In: Scoliosis: Causes, Symptoms and Treatment ISBN: 978-1-62081-007-1
Editors: A. Bessette et al. © 2012 Nova Science Publishers, Inc.

Chapter VI

Effects of Load Carriage on Children with Scoliosis[*]

Daniel Hung-kay Chow[†] and Alon Lai
Department of Health Technology and Informatics
The Hong Kong Polytechnic University, Hong Kong, PR China

Abstract

Scoliosis is a lateral spinal deformity. Despite extensive research, the etiology of scoliosis is still unclear. However, abnormal external loading is known to be one of the possible factors that may exacerbate the deformity. As load carriage is common for schoolchildren, it has been a concern whether an 'overweight' schoolbag would impose abnormal biomechanical and physiological stress on the spine. A series of investigations were conducted to compare the effects of backpack carriage on pulmonary function, standing posture and balance as well as gait performance in children with and without scoliosis. Pulmonary function and balance control in both standing and walking were found to be adversely affected by increased backpack weight. The effects of backpack carriage on children with and without scoliosis were similar.

---

[*] A version of this chapter also appears in Load Carriage in School Children: Epidemiology and Exercise Science, edited by Youlian Hong, published by Nova Science Publishers, Inc. It was submitted for appropriate modifications in an effort to encourage wider dissemination of research.
[†] Corresponding email: *Daniel.Chow@inet.polyu.edu.hk.*

However, pulmonary function and stability control of children with scoliosis were consistently poorer than normal. The results of these studies showed that the limit of backpack weight recommended for normal children based on the changes in biomechanical and physiological measures might not be applicable for those with scoliosis. However, there is still a lack of evidence whether carrying backpack would accelerate curve progression in children with scoliosis. Further investigation is warranted to address this question.

Keywords: Load Carriage, Scoliosis, Pulmonary Function, Posture and Balance, Gait

Introduction

Adolescent Idiopathic Scoliosis

Scoliosis is a lateral spinal deformity often coupled with vertebral rotation. Most of the cases are idiopathic with prevalence of about 2-4% of children [1,2]. Although scoliosis is a deformity of the spine, it has been demonstrated to affect the pulmonary function, standing balance and gait performance of children with scoliosis.

a) Pulmonary Function

For children with scoliosis, the chest wall will usually be distorted and the respiratory and cardiovascular systems will also be affected if the thoracic spine is involved [3]. Therefore, the effect of scoliosis on pulmonary function has been a concern. Gazioglu et al. [4] found that the pulmonary function of children with scoliosis was adversely affected with reduced vital capacity, total lung capacity, maximum expiratory flow, maximum mid-expiratory flow and peak flow rate. They found that the pulmonary impairments could be improved after surgical correction of the scoliosis. Restrictive pulmonary function with decreased diffusing capacity, arterial oxygen tension, ventilatory response to carbon dioxide, vital capacity and total lung capacity was also observed in the studies by Weber et al. [5], Muirhead and Conner [6] and Boyer et al. [7]. Moreover, both Weber et al. [5] and Muirhead and Conner [6] demonstrated that the severity of pulmonary dysfunction was associated with the degree of scoliosis. Upadhyay et al. [8] and Takahashi et al. [9] further investigated the association between the respiratory function and the severity of spinal deformity. Upadhyay et al. [8] showed that Cobb angle, vertebral rotation and vertebral rotation flexibility were significantly associated with vital capacity and forced vital capacity, while the severity of kyphotic deformation was significantly correlated with lung residual volume, total capacity and functional residual capacity as well as the forced expiratory flow from 25%-75% of forced vital capacity (FEF_{25-75}). Takahashi et al. [9] demonstrated that the reduced lung vital capacity in scoliotic adolescents was correlated with the sagittal diameter of the thoracic cage, the total lung area and the vertebral rotation at T8 and T9 levels.

b) Standing Balance

Standing balance has been used to study the general motor control of an individual. During upright stance, the postural muscles of the trunk and lower limbs are coordinated to maintain the body equilibrium by controlling the body center of gravity (CG) within its stability limits and prevent the body from collapsing due to the gravity. The activation of the postural muscles is mainly governed by the peripheral inputs from the visual, somatosensory and vestibular systems to detect the position and movement of the body in space with respect to the gravity. Thus, the body is not static but sways within an invisible boundary during upright stance [10].

The standing balance of an individual is usually quantified by measuring the body sway with the aids of a force platform. Sahlstrand et al. [11] compared the body sway of children with and without scoliosis during upright stance. They found that the children with scoliosis had larger sagittal sway, lateral sway and total sway area compared to the normal. Similar results were reported by Byl and Gray [12], Byl et al. [13], Chen et al. [14] and Nault et al. [15]. Additionally, Byl and Gray [12], Byl et al. [13] and Chen et al. [14] found that the balance control of children with scoliosis was further deteriorated when their visual and/or somatosensory inputs were challenged particularly for the children with larger deformity. Nault et al. [15] studied the differences in motion between the center of pressure (COP) and center of mass (COM) and found that children with scoliosis required greater neuromuscular demand for maintaining their standing balance. Lenke et al. [16] demonstrated the impaired balance control associated with scoliosis was improved after surgical correction, particularly in the coronal plane. These studies revealed that children with scoliosis have poorer standing balance than normal especially in the coronal plane. The differences become more apparent when the afferent inputs are challenged.

c) Gait Performance

A deficiency in static balance control may affect the dynamic performance of children with scoliosis. The effect of scoliosis on gait performance has therefore, been studied. Barrack et al. [17] compared the gait kinematics between children with and without scoliosis and found that the children with scoliosis tried to increase their gait stability by reducing their walking velocity, stride length and single limb support time. Chen et al. [14] and Mahaudens et al. [18,19] also reported similar change in gait pattern for children with scoliosis. Giakas et al. [20] found that the poorer stability mainly occurred during the stance phase. Mahaudens et al. [18,19] found that the demand on children with scoliosis in walking was higher evidenced by lower efficiency in transforming between the gravitational potential energy and the kinetic energy for locomotion. They also suggested that the modified gait with lower walking efficiency might be associated with the restricted pelvic and hip motion resulting from prolonged activation of the bilateral spinal and pelvic muscles. On the other hand, Schizas et al. [21], Chockalingam et al. [22] and Kramers-de Quervain et al. [23] found that the gait symmetry of children with scoliosis was also affected with asymmetric left and right ground reaction force during walking. However, the asymmetry was found to be independent of curve direction, curve magnitude and vertebral rotation. These studies implied that children with scoliosis have asymmetric gait with poor stability and this is compensated by reducing the single limb supporting time and walking speed.

Backpack Carriage

Backpack carriage is common in children for carrying books, stationeries and personal belongings to and from schools. The effects of backpack carriage on the pulmonary function, gait, standing posture and balance of children have been widely investigated.

a) Pulmonary Function

Lai and Jones [24] studied the effects of backpack carriage with different weights on the pulmonary function of normal primary schoolchildren. They found that when carrying a backpack of 20% or 30% of the children's body weight (BW), the lung volume was restricted with decreased forced expiratory volume in the first second (FEV_1) and forced vital capacity (FVC), which was not seen when the children carried a backpack of 10% BW. They also observed similar change when the participants adopted a kyphotic standing posture even without carrying any load. Li et al. [25] found that there was no obvious change in respiratory characteristics for 10-year-old children walking with backpack of 10% BW. However, when the backpack weight was increased to 15% or 20% BW, a more rapid breathing frequency was detected. They also demonstrated that there were linear relationships among backpack weight, breathing frequency and trunk inclination. These studies revealed that carrying a backpack heavier than 10% BW would have a restrictive effect on lung capacity and increase the respiratory demand.

b) Standing Posture and Balance

During backpack carriage, the backpack load tends to shift the body centre of gravity (CG) posteriorly. In order to maintain the body equilibrium, the spinal curvature and body posture have to be modified so as to maintain the COP within the base of support. Chow et al. [26], Devroey et al. [27] and Negrini and Negrini [28] showed that when children carrying a backpack, there was an increase in trunk forward inclination with lumbar flexion and anterior pelvic tilt. The cervical spine was found to adopt an extended posture so as to compensate for the forward inclined trunk while preserving the vision to the front. The contribution of the thoracic spine to backpack carriage was however, not consistent. Devroey et al. [22] demonstrated an increase in thoracic kyphosis, while Chow et al. [26] and Negrini and Negrini [28] found a reduction in thoracic kyphosis during backpack carriage. Nault et al. [15] showed that standing posture was associated with standing stability mainly in the sagittal plane. As backpack carriage primarily affects the standing posture in the sagittal plane, the standing stability is probably affected. Zultowski and Aruin [29] compared the static standing balance of children between loaded and unloaded conditions and found that when the children carried a backpack, their body swayed faster and farther with the magnitudes of change associated with the backpack weight. Apart from studying the effect on static standing balance, Palumbo et al. [30] found that backpack carriage also resulted in a decrease in dynamic stability with decreased velocity and accuracy in moving the body to the desired positions mainly in the sagittal plane. All these studies showed that both the standing posture and balance are adversely affected by backpack carriage particularly in the sagittal plane.

c) Gait Performance

Pascoe et al. [31] found that walking with a backpack significantly increased trunk forward inclination with decreased stride length. Increased trunk inclination with backpack weight was also reported by Hong and

Brueggemann [32], Goodgold et al. [33], Hong and Cheung [34], Li et al. [25] and Singh and Koh [35]. Moreover, Hong and Cheung [34] and Li et al. [25] showed that the trunk inclination was associated with the carrying time and it was probably resulted from the fatigue of the trapezius muscle which was responsible for counterbalancing the backpack load [36]. As the trapezius is a major trunk extensor [37], its fatigue may lead to upper trunk flexion and consequently resulted in forward trunk inclination. In response to the forward inclined trunk, the cervical spine had to extend so as to maintain the gaze to the front [38] and the change of cervical extension was associated with the backpack weight and carrying duration. Moreover, Hong and Brueggemann [32], Wang et al. [39], Cottalorda et al. [40] and Singh and Koh [35] also showed that the gait temporal-distance parameters were affected when walking with a backpack. These included increased double support time and stance duration together with decreased walking speed, cadence, stride length, single support time and swing duration. The walking stability was probability maintained by the increased double support time and stance duration. Singh and Koh [35] further studied the effect of backpack vertical position on gait and found that there was a trend to have more obvious changes in gait temporal-distance parameters when a backpack was carried at the lower back (i.e. inferior to T8-T9).

In summary, both scoliosis and backpack carriage have been separately demonstrated to compromise the pulmonary function, standing posture and balance as well as the gait performance of children. However, it was still not clear whether there was any interaction between these two factors. A series of studies were therefore, conducted to fill in this knowledge gap.

Methods

Pulmonary Function

The pulmonary functions of schoolgirls with and without scoliosis in carrying backpack of different weights were compared [41]. Seventeen girls with moderate scoliosis (Cobb angle between 26° and 50°) and 18 girls with normal musculoskeletal development were recruited. Spirometric characteristics including force vital capacity (FVC), forced expiratory volume in the first second (FEV_1), ratio of FEV_1 to FVC, peak expiratory flow (PEF) and forced expiratory flow during the middle half of the expiration ($FEF_{25-75\%}$) of the participants were measured when the participants were asked to maintain a normal erect stance with or without carrying a double-strap backpack of different weights (i.e. 5%, 7.5%, 10%, 12.5% or 15% of their body weight (BW)). The centre of gravity (CG) of the backpack was positioned between T11 and T12 level. The participants were instructed to take several normal breaths, inspire completely, and finally exhale as hard and fast as possible for 6 seconds or a 3-second of plateau was observed. Totally, three measurement trials were performed and the variation of expiratory volume between trials was controlled within 0.2L.

Standing Posture and Balance

The effects of scoliosis and backpack carriage on standing posture and balance of schoolgirls were evaluated [42]. Twenty-six schoolgirls with mild scoliosis (Cobb angle ranged from 10° to 25°) and 20 age-matched normal girls were recruited. All the girls were asked to stand with or without carrying a standardized dual-strap backpack of 7.5%, 10%, 12.5% or 15% BW. The CG of the backpack was located between T11 and T12 level. During the measurement, the participants were asked to maintain a relaxed erect stance for 90 seconds with the arms freely positioning at the sides and the gaze fixed on a reference point located at 2m in the front at eye level. The standing posture was measured using a motion analysis system (Vicon 370, Oxford Metrics, Oxford, UK) to determine the kinematics of the head, trunk and pelvis in three anatomical planes. The standing balance was measured simultaneously using a force platform (AMTI, Newton, MA, USA) to quantify the sway of the body from the mean position in both the antero-posterior (AP) and medio-lateral (ML) directions.

Gait Performance

The gait patterns of schoolgirls with and without scoliosis during backpack carriage of different weights were compared [43]. Twenty-two normal girls and 28 age-matched girls with mild scoliosis (Cobb angle between 10° and 25°) participated in the study. The gait temporal-distance characteristics as well as the kinematics and kinetics of the hip, knee and ankles joints were determined using a motion analysis system (Vicon 370, Oxford Metrics, Oxford, UK) and two force platforms (AMTI, Newton, MA, USA). The girls were instructed to walk with barefoot at natural cadence along a 10 m walkway with or without carrying a backpack of 7.5%, 10%, 12.5% or 15% BW (Figure 1). Three complete gait cycles were obtained for each condition and the data were averaged for data analysis.

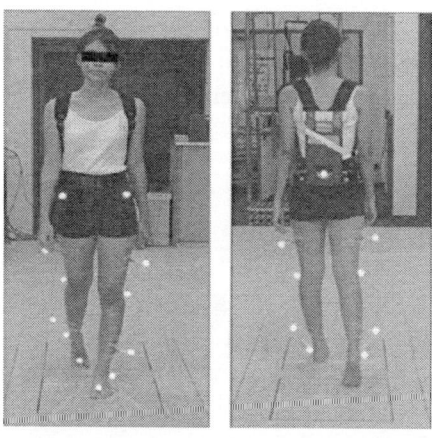

Figure 1. A schoolgirl walked along a 10m walkway with a backpack. Two force platforms and a motion analysis system with the aids of reflective markers were used to determine the gait temporal-distance characteristics as well as the kinematics and kinetics of the hip, knee and ankles joints. [43]

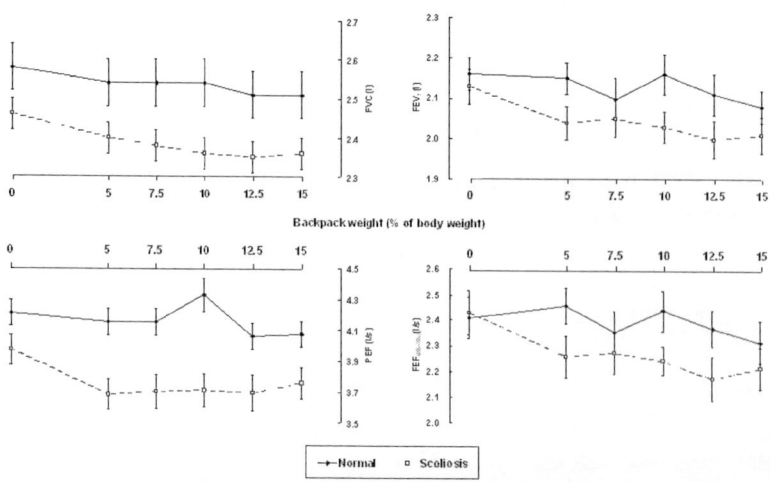

Figure 2. The changes of force vital capacity (FVC), forced expiratory volume in the first second (FEV1), ratio of FEV1 to FVC, peak expiratory flow (PEF) and forced expiratory flow during the middle half of the expiration (FEF25-75%) in girls with or without scoliosis when carrying backpack of different weights (0%, 5%, 7.5%, 10%, 12.5% or 15% of body weight). The standard error is shown as error bar. [41].

Results

Pulmonary Function

There was no interaction between the factors of backpack weight and scoliosis on the pulmonary function. The effects of backpack weight on all the measured pulmonary parameters were similar between the normal controls and the girls with scoliosis. Both FVC and FEV_1 were found to decrease with increased backpack weight. However, compared to the normal schoolgirls, FVC, FEV_1, PEF and $FEF_{25-75\%}$ of the girls with scoliosis were consistently lower (Figure 2).

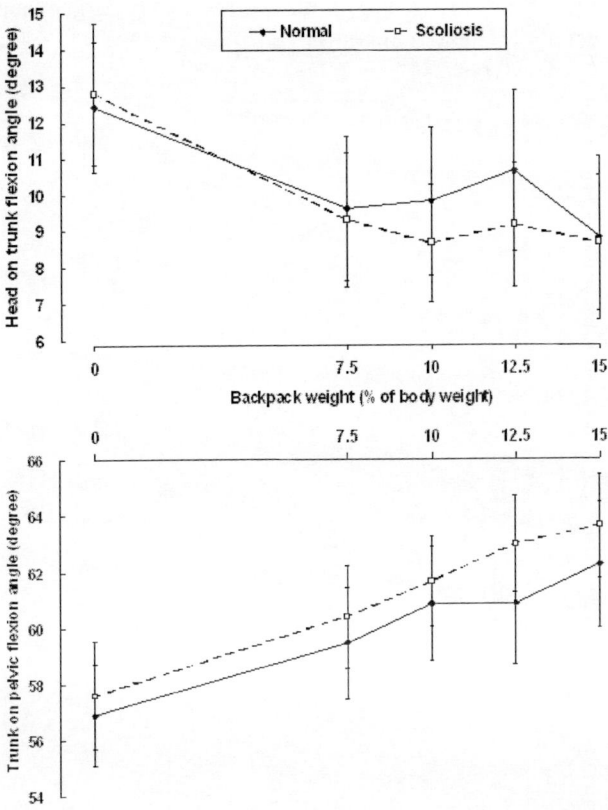

Figure 3. The changes of trunk on pelvic flexion angle and head on trunk flexion angle during upright stance for normal and scoliotic girls carrying a backpack of different weights (0%, 7.5%, 10%, 12.5% or 15% of body weight). The standard error is indicated as error bar. [42].

Standing Posture and Balance

Both the standing posture and balance of the girls with and without scoliosis were significantly affected by backpack and the magnitudes of changes were found to be associated with the backpack weight. All the participants flexed their trunk relative to the pelvis and extended their head when they carried a backpack (Figure 3). Compared to the unloaded condition, carrying a backpack of 15% BW significantly increased the range of COP motion in the AP direction. Although the standing postures adopted by the children with and without scoliosis during backpack carriage were similar, the postural control of the girls with scoliosis was found to be poorer than the normal controls. The deviations of the head and pelvic positions from their mean standing posture of the girls with scoliosis were larger than the normal controls especially in the ML direction.

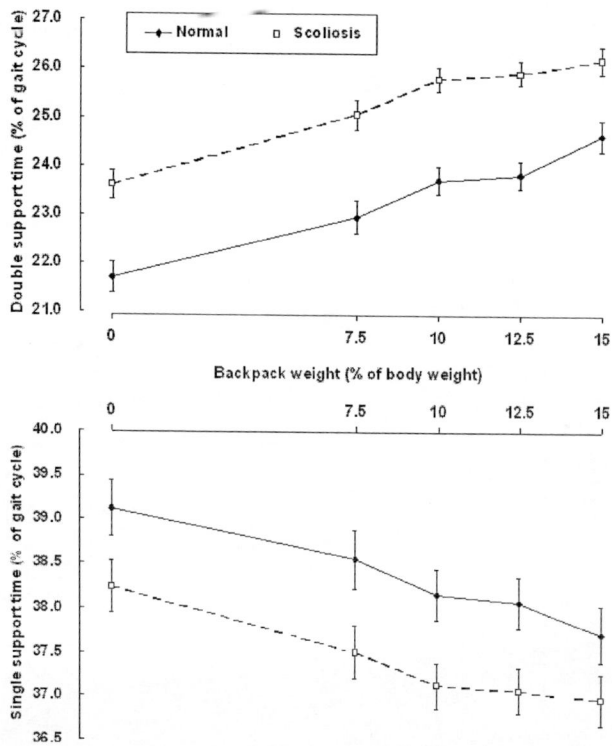

Figure 4. The changes of double support time and single support time for girls with and without scoliosis carrying a backpack of different weights (0%, 7.5%, 10%, 10%, 12.5% and 15% of body weight). The standard error is shown as error bar. [43].

Gait Performance

There was no interaction between the backpack weight and scoliosis factors on gait for all the measured parameters. Similar walking patterns were observed for both the normal controls and the girls with scoliosis for all the backpack loads. An increase in backpack weight was found to result in significantly decreased walking speed, cadence, stride length, step length, single support duration and pelvic motion as well as increased hip joint flexion-extension motion, moment and power (for both generation and absorption). Compared to the normal controls, the girls with scoliosis walked with significantly longer double support time and shorter single support time (Figure 4) as well as knee joint power generation and absorption in the sagittal plane (Figure 5).

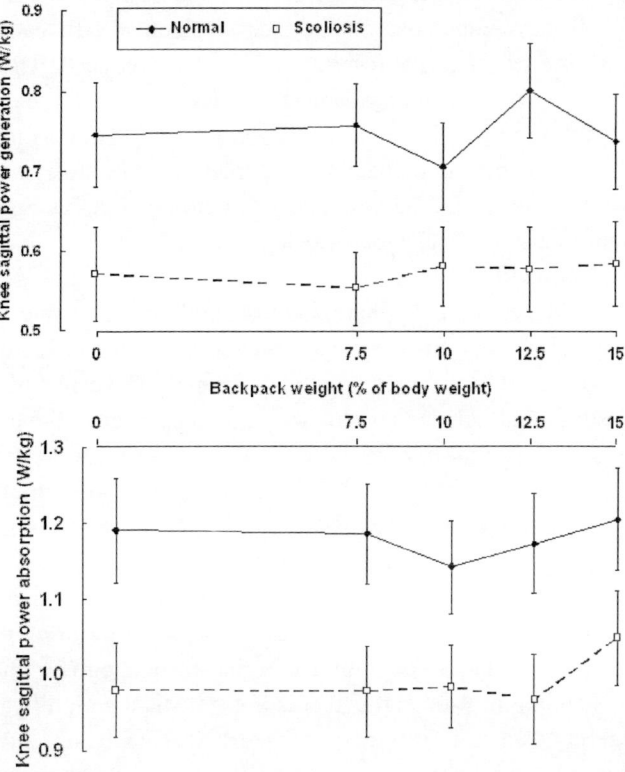

Figure 5. The changes of knee sagittal power generation and absorption for girls with and without scoliosis carrying a backpack of different weights (0%, 7.5%, 10%, 12.5% or 15% of body weight). The standard error is indicated as error bar. [43].

Discussion

Carrying a backpack was shown to induce restrictive effect for both the normal controls and the girls with scoliosis [44]. The restriction might be resulted from the backpack straps [45,46] or the change of standing posture during backpack carriage. Chow et al. [42] showed that when carrying a backpack, there was an increase in trunk forward inclination for maintaining the body equilibrium. Although the changes of curvatures at different spinal regions have not been documented in children with scoliosis, Devroey et al. [27] suggested that the forward trunk inclination observed in girls with and without scoliosis was resulted from the anterior pelvic tilt coupled with flexion of lumbar and thoracic spine. Both FVC and FEV_1 have been demonstrated to be significantly decreased when standing with a kyphotic posture even without carrying any load [24]. When a kyphotic posture is adopted, the chest muscles might be in a disadvantage position and their mechanical efficiency and power in controlling the rib cage for respiration might be reduced. The interaction between the factors of scoliosis and backpack weight on the pulmonary function of children was not found to be significant [41]. This indicated that the physiological demands of backpack carriage and scoliosis on girls were additive. In other words, as the pulmonary function of girls with scoliosis was poorer than normal, backpack carriage would further increase their physiological demand.

It was interested to note that although both the standing posture and balance were apparently affected by scoliosis and backpack carriage, their effects were different in different anatomical planes. The effect of scoliosis on standing postural and balance control was more apparent in the coronal plane while the effect of backpack carriage was more apparent in the sagittal plane. Moreover, gait analysis showed that the gait stability of normal girls was better than the girls with scoliosis. When carrying a backpack, both the normal controls and the girls with scoliosis walked slower with decreased cadence, stride length, step length and single support duration. The demand for walking was elevated with increased joint flexion-extension motion, moment and power of the hip joints. The interaction between scoliosis and backpack carriage on standing posture and gait was not statistically significant, standing and gait stability were relatively poorer for girls with scoliosis.

Bracing (thoraco-lumbo-sacral orthosis) is a common non-invasive treatment for patients with scoliosis for preventing further progression of scoliosis. It is natural to expect that children with scoliosis will be wearing a brace in additional to carrying a backpack. The effects of bracing have also been shown to adversely affect the standing balance of children with scoliosis when carrying a backpack and standing on an unstable surface [47]. As bracing is a rigid orthotic treatment which applies corrective forces to the spine and usually covers the spine from the thoracic to the sacral regions, the pulmonary function of children with scoliosis may further be affected. Future study is therefore, required to determine the significance of the bracing effect. The effects of other factors should be considered in future studies. All the studies were conducted for children with mild or moderate scoliosis (Cobb angle of 10°-25° and 26°-50°), the findings might not be applicable for children with severe scoliosis (>50°). Additionally, all measurements were performed immediately after putting on a backpack. As schoolchildren usually have to carry their backpack for a period of time for daily travel [48], the long-term effects of backpack carriage on children with scoliosis should also be investigated.

Other carrying methods, such as carrying over one shoulder, front pack, double pack and one-strap athletic shoulder bag, are also commonly used. The effects of these carrying methods have also been shown to affect trunk inclination, spinal curvature and trunk muscle activity [49,50] and symmetric load carriage is usually recommended. However, as scoliosis is a lateral deformity of the spine, it is still not certain whether an asymmetric applied load might accelerate curve progression in scoliosis, or on the other way round, it could be used to slow down the curve progression if the load and position are properly controlled. Further study in this area is warranted.

Conclusion

The pulmonary function, standing balance and gait stability were found to be significantly affected by both scoliosis and backpack carriage without any significant interactive effect. Increased backpack weight was shown to significantly increase the biomechanical and physiological demand for both children with and without scoliosis. As children with scoliosis have generally lower performance than normal, the limit of backpack weight recommended for normal children based on the changes observed in various biomechanical and physiological parameters should not be suitable for children with scoliosis. However, there is still a lack of evidence whether backpack carriage would accelerate curve progress or not. Further biomechanical study of the direct effect of load carriage on the children's spine with deformity would be needed. Moreover, further investigation on the effect of bracing, severity of scoliosis, carrying duration and methods would be useful to provide additional knowledge of the effects of backpack carriage for children with scoliosis.

References

[1] Kane, W. J. and Moe, J. H. (1970). A scoliosis-prevalence survey in Minnesota. *Clin. Orthop. Relat. Res.* 69:216-8.
[2] Rogala, E. J., Drummond, D. S. and Gurr, J. (1978). Scoliosis: incidence and natural history. A prospective epidemiological study. *J. Bone Joint Surg. Am.* 60:173-176.
[3] Koumbourlis, A. C. (2006). Scoliosis and the respiratory system. *Paediatr. Respir. Rev.* 7:152-160.
[4] Gazioglu, K., Goldstein, L. A., Femi-Pearse, D. and Yu, P. N. (1968). Pulmonary function in idiopathic scoliosis: Comparative evaluation before and after orthopaedic correction. *J. Bone Joint Surg. Am.* 50: 1391-1399.
[5] Weber, B., Smith, J. P., Briscoe, W. A., Friedman, S. A. and King, T. K. (1975). Pulmonary function in asymptomatic adolescents with idiopathic scoliosis. *Am. Rev. Respir. Dis.* 111:389-97.
[6] Muirhead, A. and Conner, A. N. (1985). The assessment of lung function in children with scoliosis. *J. Bone Joint Surg. Br.* 67:699-702.
[7] Boyer, J., Amin, N., Taddonio, R. and Dozor, A. J. (1996). Evidence of airway obstruction in children with idiopathic scoliosis. *Chest* 109: 1532-1535.
[8] Upadhyay, S. S., Mullaji, A. B., Luk, K. D. and Leong, J. C. (1995). Relation of spinal and thoracic cage deformities and their flexibilities with altered pulmonary functions in adolescent idiopathic scoliosis. *Spine* 20:2415-2420.
[9] Takahashi, S., Suzuki, N., Asazuma, T., Kono, K., Ono, T. and Toyama, Y. (2007). Factors of thoracic cage deformity that affect pulmonary function in adolescent idiopathic thoracic scoliosis. *Spine* 32:106-112.
[10] Shumway-Cook, A. and Woollacott, M. H. (2001). *Motor contro: theory and practical applications* (2nd). Baltimore, MD: Lippincott Williams and Wilkins.
[11] Sahlstrand, T., Ortengren, R. and Nachemson, A. (1978). Postural equilibrium in adolescent idiopathic scoliosis. *Acta Orthop. Scand.* 49:354-365.

[12] Byl, N. N. and Gray, J. M. (1993). Complex balance reactions in different sensory conditions: adolescents with and without idiopathic scoliosis. *J. Orthop. Res.* 11: 215-227.

[13] Byl, N. N., Holland, S., Jurek, A. and Hu, S. S. (1997). Postural imbalance and vibratory sensitivity in patients with idiopathic scoliosis: implications for treatment. *J. Orthop. Sports Phys. Ther.* 26:60-68.

[14] Chen, P. Q., Wang, J. L., Tsuang, Y. H., Liao, T. L., Huang, P. I. and Hang, Y. S. (1998). The postural stability control and gait pattern of idiopathic scoliosis adolescents. *Clin. Biomech.* (Bristol, Avon) 13: S52-S58.

[15] Nault, M. L., Allard, P., Hinse, S., Le Blanc, R., Caron, O., Labelle, H. and Sadeghi, H. (2002). Relations between standing stability and body posture parameters in adolescent idiopathic scoliosis. *Spine* 27: 1911-1917.

[16] Lenke, L. G., Engsberg, J. R., Ross, S. A., Reitenbach, A., Blanke, K. and Bridwell, K. H. (2001). Prospective dynamic functional evaluation of gait and spinal balance following spinal fusion in adolescent idiopathic scoliosis. *Spine* 26: E330-337.

[17] Barrack, R. L., Whitecloud, T. S., 3rd, Burke, S. W., Cook, S. D. and Harding, A. F. (1984). Proprioception in idiopathic scoliosis. *Spine* (Phila Pa 1976) 9:681-685.

[18] Mahaudens, P., Banse, X., Mousny, M. and Detrembleur, C. (2009). Gait in adolescent idiopathic scoliosis: kinematics and electromyographic analysis. *Eur. Spine J.* 18: 512-521.

[19] Mahaudens, P., Thonnard, J. L. and Detrembleur, C. (2005). Influence of structural pelvic disorders during standing and walking in adolescents with idiopathic scoliosis. *Spine J* 5:427-433.

[20] Giakas, G., Baltzopoulos, V., Dangerfield, P. H., Dorgan, J. C. and Dalmira, S. (1996). Comparison of gait patterns between healthy and scoliotic patients using time and frequency domain analysis of ground reaction forces. *Spine* 21:2235-2242.

[21] 21. asymmetries in patients with idiopathic scoliosis using vertical forces measurement only. *Eur. Spine J.* 7:95-8.

[22] Chockalingam, N., Dangerfield, P. H., Rahmatalla, A., Ahmed el, N. and Cochrane, T. (2004). Assessment of ground reaction force during scoliotic gait. *Eur. Spine J.* 13: 750-754.

[23] Kramers-de Quervain, I. A., Muller, R., Stacoff, A., Grob, D. and Stussi, E. (2004). Gait analysis in patients with idiopathic scoliosis. *Eur. Spine J.* 13:449-456.

[24] Lai, J. P. and Jones, A. Y. (2001). The effect of shoulder-girdle loading by a school bag on lung volumes in Chinese primary school children. *Early Hum. Dev.* 62:79-86.

[25] Li, J. X., Hong, Y. and Robinson, P. D. (2003). The effect of load carriage on movement kinematics and respiratory parameters in children during walking. *Eur. J. Appl. Physiol.* 90:35-43.

[26] Chow, D. H., Leung, K. T. and Holmes, A. D. (2007b). Changes in spinal curvature and proprioception of schoolboys carrying different weights of backpack. *Ergonomics* 50:2148-2156.

[27] Devroey, C., Jonkers, I., de Becker, A., Lenaerts, G. and Spaepen, A. (2007). Evaluation of the effect of backpack load and position during standing and walking using biomechanical, physiological and subjective measures. *Ergonomics* 50:728-742.

[28] Negrini, S. and Negrini, A. (2007). Postural effects of symmetrical and asymmetrical loads on the spines of schoolchildren. *Scoliosis* 2:8.

[29] Zultowski, I. and Arum, A. (2008). Carrying loads and postural sway in standing: the effect of load placement and magnitude. *Work* 30:359-68.

[30] Palumbo, N., George, B., Johnson, A. and Cade, D. (2001). The effects of backpack load carrying on dynamic balance as measured by limits of stability. *Work* 16:123-129.

[31] Pascoe, D. D., Pascoe, D. E., Wang, Y. T., Shim, D. M. and Kim, C. K. (1997). Influence of carrying book bags on gait cycle and posture of youths. *Ergonomics* 40: 631-641.

[32] Hong, Y. and Brueggemann, G. P. (2000). Changes in gait patterns in 10-year-old boys with increasing loads when walking on a treadmill. *Gait Posture* 11:254-259.

[33] Goodgold, S., Mohr, K., Samant, A., Parke, T., Burns, T. and Gardner, L. (2002). Effects of backpack load and task demand on trunk forward lean: Pilot findings on two boys. *Work* 18:213-220.

[34] Hong, Y. and Cheung, C. K. (2003). Gait and posture responses to backpack load during level walking in children. *Gait Posture* 17:28-33.

[35] Singh, T. and Koh, M. (2009). Effects of backpack load position on spatiotemporal parameters and trunk forward lean. *Gait Posture* 29: 49-53.

[36] Hong, Y., Li, J. X. and Fong, D. T. (2008). Effect of prolonged walking with backpack loads on trunk muscle activity and fatigue in children. *J. Electromyogr Kinesiol* 18(6):990-996.

[37] Konrad, P., Schmitz, K. and Denner, A. (2001). Neuromuscular Evaluation of Trunk-Training Exercises. *J. Athl. Train.* 36:109-118.

[38] Chansirinukor, W., Wilson, D., Grimmer, K. and Dansie, B. (2001). Effects of backpacks on students: measurement of cervical and shoulder posture. *Aust. J. Physiother.* 47:110-116.

[39] Wang, Y., Pascoe, D. D. and Weimar, W. (2001). Evaluation of book backpack load during walking. *Ergonomics* 44:858-69.

[40] Cottalorda, J., Rahmani, A., Diop, M., Gautheron, V., Ebermeyer, E. and Belli, A. (2003). Influence of school bag carrying on gait kinetics. *J. Pediatr. Orthop. B.* 12: 357-364.

[41] Chow, D. H., Ng, X. H., Holmes, A. D., Cheng, J. C., Yao, F. Y. and Wong, M. S. (2005). Effects of backpack loading on the pulmonary capacities of normal schoolgirls and those with adolescent idiopathic scoliosis. *Spine* 30:E649-654.

[42] Chow, D. H., Kwok, M. L., Cheng, J. C., Lao, M. L., Holmes, A. D., Au-Yang, A., Yao, F. Y. and Wong, M. S. (2006b). The effect of backpack weight on the standing posture and balance of schoolgirls with adolescent idiopathic scoliosis and normal controls. *Gait. Posture* 24:173-181.

[43] Chow, D. H., Kwok, M. L., Au-Yang, A. C., Holmes, A. D., Cheng, J. C., Yao, F. Y. and Wong, M. S. (2006a). The effect of load carriage on the gait of girls with adolescent idiopathic scoliosis and normal controls. *Med. Eng. Phys.* 28:430-437.

[44] Ruppel, G. (2009). *Manual of pulmonary function testing* (9th). St. Louis, Mo.: Mosby Elsevier.

[45] Bygrave, S., Legg, S. J., Myers, S. and Llewellyn, M. (2004). Effect of backpack fit on lung function. *Ergonomics* 47:324-329.

[46] Legg, S. J. and Cruz, C. O. (2004). Effect of single and double strap backpacks on lung function. *Ergonomics* 47:318-23.

[47] Chow, D. H., Leung, D. S. and Holmes, A. D. (2007a). The effects of load carriage and bracing on the balance of schoolgirls with adolescent idiopathic scoliosis. *Eur. Spine J.* 16:1351-1358.

[48] Haselgrove, C., Straker, L., Smith, A., O'Sullivan, P., Perry, M. and Sloan, N. (2008). Perceived school bag load, duration of carriage, and method of transport to school are associated with spinal pain in adolescents: an observational study. *Aust. J. Physiother.* 54:193-200.

[49] Fiolkowski, P., Horodyski, M., Bishop, M., Williams, M. and Stylianou, L. (2006). Changes in gait kinematics and posture with the use of a front pack. *Ergonomics* 49: 885-894.

[50] Motmans, R. R., Tomlow, S. and Vissers, D. (2006). Trunk muscle activity in different modes of carrying schoolbags. *Ergonomics* 49:127-138.

In: Scoliosis: Causes, Symptoms and Treatment   ISBN: 978-1-62081-007-1
Editors: A. Bessette et al.   © 2012 Nova Science Publishers, Inc.

Chapter VII

The Pineal Gland, Melatonin and Scoliosis[*]

Gregory Day[†] *and Bruce McPhee*
University of Queensland, Brisbane, Australia

Abstract

Over the past 25 years, chicken studies implicated experimental pinealectomy as acause of scoliosis. The nature of the scoliosis was demonstrated to be similar to that of human idiopathic scoliosis. Subsequent research involved a primate (Rhesus monkey) experimental pinealectomy model. Scoliosis was not induced by pinealectomy. In a recent Australian study, no causal link was established between pineal lesions and the development of idiopathic scoliosis. Melatonin is the only known hormone secreted by the pineal gland in humans. Previous research concluded that melatonin secretion was similar in those with idiopathic scoliosis and aged-matched controls. A recent Korean study concluded that permanent melatonin deficiency was not a causative factor in the aetiology of (AIS) adolescent idiopathic scoliosis. Over a period of

---

[*] A version of this chapter also appears in The Pineal Gland and Melatonin: Recent Advances in Development, Imaging, Disease and Treatment, edited by Mehmet Turgut and Raj Kumar, published by Nova Science Publishers, Inc. It was submitted for appropriate modifications in an effort to encourage wider dissemination of research.

[†] Correspondence: Gregory Day, MD, Professor, Level 5, St Andrew's Place, 33 North Street, Spring Hill, Queensland, Australia 4000. E-mail: *ggandlda@bigpond.net.au*.

25 years, research involving the production of scoliosis following pinealectomy in small animal models has not been reproducible in the human model. The search for a scientifically sound human model to investigate the etiology of idiopathic scoliosis continues.

Introduction

The existence of the pineal gland was postulated nearly two millennia ago. It was not until 1958 that discovery of the active pineal hormone, melatonin, opened the way into researching the functions of the pineal gland [1,2]. Subsequently, Axelrod was able to elucidate the biochemical cascade for the synthesis of melatonin in the pinealocytes [3]. The pineal gland's anatomical location and function are now established. It is known to exert a physiological effect through a variety of actions such as an endocrine gland, a transducer, and a regulator of hormones and as a damped circadian oscillator. Melatonin is thought or known to mediate all of these functions. Animal research has demonstrated a relationship between the production of melatonin and the modulation of circadian rhythm and sleep regulation. In addition, melatonin is suspected of influencing reproductive physiology, cardiovascular function, immunological regulation, and psychiatric disorders. It is not clear to what extent the results from animal studies can be extrapolated to humans. Perhaps one of the most unusual and unexpected findings is the relationship between the pineal gland, melatonin and scoliosis in experimental animals.

Experimental Scoliosis – Pinealectomy and Melatonin

Research involving the production of experimental scoliosis in chickens and rodents commenced following a serendipitous experiment in France 40 years ago [4].

Experimental pinealectomy in three-day-old white leghorn chickens of both genders led to the development of thoracic scoliosis, [5] whereas a sham procedure did not [6]. Between 50 and 100% of pinealectomized chickens developed scoliosis [4,6]. The prevalence of scoliosis in chickens pinealectomized between 2 and 18 days after hatching was not significantly different [7]. However, scoliosis was only occasionally observed after older chickens underwent experimental pinealectomy [8]. The critical step involved removing the entire pineal gland and/or stalk [9,10]. The induced scoliosis appeared to be similar to human idiopathic scoliosis [11,12]. However, angular thoracic scoliosis was also observed in some pinealectomized chickens as well as controls [11,13,14]. Intra-muscular auto-transplantation of the pineal gland into pinealectomized chickens prevented the scoliosis developing in 90%, [12] but the results of this research were subsequently repudiated [15,16].

Melatonin (N-acetyl-5-methoxytryptamine) is the only known hormone secreted by the poultry pineal gland [17]. Pinealectomy on three-day-old chickens resulted in reduced melatonin levels and elimination of the melatonin circadian rhythm [18]. Although a low serum melatonin level was reported to be associated with scoliosis in pinealectomized chickens, [18] other researchers were unable to validate the association [7,19]. Induced melatonin suppression by constant light resulted in the development of scoliosis in 15% of white Leghorn chickens, [20] but it had no effect on Nihon chickens [21]. Intra-peritoneal injections of melatonin (2.5 mg/100 mg body weight) into pinealectomized white Leghorn chickens for a period of three weeks prevented scoliosis in 80% [18], but injections of melatonin (2.5 mg/1 kg body weight) had no effect on pinealectomized Mountain Hubbard chickens [22]. The latter dose was believed to restore melatonin levels to a more physiological range. Daily intra-peritoneal injections of 5-hydroxy-l-tryptophan (a precursor of both serotonin and melatonin) into white Leghorn pinealectomized chickens retarded scoliosis development in 30% [23]. Pinealectomy in young chickens resulted in a loss of diurnal variation in serum melatonin levels and a reduction in melatonin receptor affinity whether or not scoliosis developed. Low melatonin levels and reduced spinal cord melatonin binding were believed to be not the sole factors in the etiology of scoliosis in pinealectomized chickens [24].

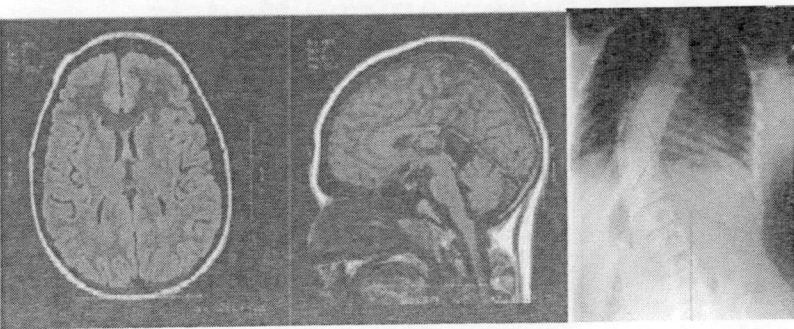

Figure 1. (a) Magnetic resonance images of the brain of a 12-year-old male with a pineal cyst. (b) Plain AP radiograph demonstrating his right thoracic scoliosis.

Other experimental animal pinealectomy models (e.g., hamsters) also produced scoliosis [25]. Scoliosis did not develop in pinealectomized quadrupedal rats but developed in all pinealectomized bipedal male Sprague-Dawley rats, implying a postural mechanism [26]. Scoliosis was observed in 64% of a bipedal model of a strain of mouse that exhibited depressed melatonin levels in plasma and the pineal gland, including some with double curves, after 40 weeks [27]. Bipedal ambulation in a standard mouse was associated with scoliosis in only 25%, all with single curves. When combined with pinealectomy, the incidence of scoliosis in the bipedal standard mouse increased to 70%, some with double curves, comparable with bipedal melatonin-deficient mice. Daily intraperitoneal injections of melatonin prevented the development of scoliosis in the bipedal model of the melatonin-deficient mouse and pinealectomized standard mouse [28]. Hence, melatonin deficiency in bipedal mice appeared to play significant role in the development of scoliosis. Scoliosis did not develop in young pinealectomized Rhesus monkeys with a mean follow-up of 28 (range 10 to 41) months [29]. Because none of the monkeys developed scoliosis, it was postulated that the aetiological factors leading to scoliosis in lower animals may differ from idiopathic scoliosis in primates.

Pineal tumours and related conditions in humans are rare [30-33], including the case of a girl with a hypothalamic hamartoma and precocious puberty having melatonin levels low for her chronological age but appropriate for her pubertal status [34]. Scoliosis following pineal ablation in children has been reported in only one patient (Figure 1) [35-38].

Anatomic Similarities and Differences between Animal Models and Idiopathic Scoliosis

The scoliosis resulting from experimental pinealectomy in chickens and various bipedal animal models is believed to be similar to human idiopathic scoliosis. Chicken scoliosis is three-dimensional, involving rotation of the thoracic spine, producing a rib hump [39]. Single and double curves occur in both chicken and human scoliosis. The vertebral bodies in chicken and human idiopathic thoracic scoliosis are laterally wedged at the apex of the curve [13,40,41]. The vertebral wedging may result from anatomic changes in the vertebral growth plates [42]. Differential pressures on the quadrants of the vertebral growth plates can lead to the anatomic changes [42,43].

However, anatomic differences between normal human and chicken spines might overshadow the comparison of the scoliosis [6,39]. Most lumbar and thoracic vertebrae in chickens spontaneously fuse with spinal growth [39], whilst human vertebrae do not fuse. In chickens, the thoracic spine is naturally lordotic, whilst in humans, it is kyphotic. Moreover, the presence of thoracic hypokyphosis or lordosis is believed to be significant in the pathogenesis of the deformity of idiopathic thoracic scoliosis [44]. Plain imaging and magnetic resonance imaging studies of idiopathic scoliosis support a theory that relative overgrowth of the anterior elements of the human spine result in thoracic hypokyphosis or lordosis [45,46]. Chicken scoliosis may have no predilection for gender or side, whilst human idiopathic scoliosis commonly occurs predominantly on the right side of female thoracic spines. Scoliosis in pinealectomized chickens is seen only in the thoracic or thoraco-lumbar spines [11,47]. Human idiopathic scoliosis can also be present in the lumbar spine.

Unilateral visual impairment did not have a significant effect on the incidence and magnitude of scoliosis of pinealectomized chickens but affected the laterality of the curves. Visually impaired chickens had a significantly higher likelihood of left thoracic curves, tending to be as frequent as the right thoracic curves, regardless of the side of blindness. By comparison, right thoracic scoliosis predominated in visually unimpaired chickens [48].

Genetic Considerations in Animal Models and Idiopathic Scoliosis

A 55 to 90% prevalence of scoliosis was observed in highly inbred white leghorn chickens [49-51]. A study of inherited scoliosis in chickens implicated three major autosomal, recessive genes with variable expression due to incomplete penetrance, the additional effect of minor modifying genes and the environment [52]. A higher incidence of severe scoliosis in the rooster was attributed to sex-influence rather than sex-linkage inheritance [53]. Scoliosis was experimentally enhanced in genetically engineered chickens by dietary means, including feeding aminonitriles or by deprivation of trace elements such as copper, vitamin B-6, or manganese [54,55]. Interestingly, serum zinc levels significantly declined eight weeks following pinealectomy in three day-old Hydro Broiler chickens [56].

Genetic studies of adolescent idiopathic scoliosis indicated that about 11% of first-degree relatives were affected, 2.4% in second-degree relatives, and 1.4% in third-degree relatives [57-59]. Monozygous twins had a high concordance rate of idiopathic scoliosis (about 73%) compared to dizygous twins [60-62]. Genetic linkages to chromosomes 6p, 10q, 18q [63], 19p13 [64], 17p11 [65], and X [66] have been reported in adolescent idiopathic scoliosis.

Melatonin and Adolescent Idiopathic Scoliosis

Adolescents [67-69] with progressive idiopathic scoliosis were observed to have reduced night-time serum levels of melatonin, although these findings have not been supported [70-73]. In some studies, methods for identifying melatonin secretion varied and included night-time and day-time serum levels as well as 24 hour urinary excretion measurements. Because the ages of scoliotic subjects varied between reports, it was postulated that melatonin levels could influence pre-menarchal scoliotic development rather than in adolescence [74]. It was recently reported that pineal gland metabolism was similar in idiopathic scoliosis patients and controls [75].

An abnormality of melatonin receptors was implicated in a study of Hereditary Lordoscoliotic Rabbits [76]. Polymorphism of melatonin 1A receptor on chromosome 4q was not linked to human idiopathic scoliosis [77,78], but polymorphism of melatonin 1B receptor was [79]. Impaired melatonin signalling was observed in human idiopathic scoliosis but melatonin receptors were reported as being normal [80]. ASMT (Acetyl-serotonin methyl-transferase) is responsible for the final phase of synthesis of melatonin [81]. The gene is located on the pseudo-autosomal region of the short arms of the X and Y chromosomes. An unpublished study demonstrated low expression of ASMT in the vertebral growth plates in congenital and idiopathic scoliosis [82]. Tryptophan hydroxylase 1 is also a critical enzyme in melatonin synthesis. Polymorphism of this gene was observed to be associated with an incidence of idiopathic scoliosis [83].

Melatonin and Calmodulin

Calmodulin is a critical mediator of cellular calcium function and a regulator of many enzymes. Melatonin binds to calmodulin with high affinity and is believed to be a calmodulin antagonist [84]. Administration of calmodulin antagonists (tamoxifen, trifluoperozine) reduced the incidence and magnitude of scoliosis in experimental pinealectomy chicken and bipedal mouse models [85,86].

Elevated platelet calmodulin levels were observed in children with progressive scoliosis [87,88]. However, genetic expression of calmodulin was significantly lower in the vertebral articular processes and the convex-side paraspinal muscles in idiopathic scoliosis patients compared to congenital scoliosis and controls [89,90]. Platelet disorders may reflect a basic cellular pathology and a secondary change attributable to the spinal curvature or the cause of the deformity. Platelets from adolescents with minimal curve scoliosis showed significantly more deviations from normal than healthy control subjects. The most frequent of these platelet anomalies did not predict curve progression at two- to 3.5-year follow-up [91]. A number of structural and functional anomalies were observed in platelets of patients with adolescent idiopathic scoliosis [92]. Subsequently, no significant differences in platelet parameters were observed between adolescent idiopathic scoliosis patients and a control group [93]. Current controversy focuses on the lack of control data and the large variability of baseline platelet morphological and biological anomalies and platelet calmodulin levels in patients with idiopathic scoliosis [94].

Melatonin, Growth and Maturation

Animal studies have shown that melatonin has a regulatory role in reproduction by down-regulating the gonadotrophin-releasing hormone gene [95-97]. Consequently, levels of melatonin and the gonadotrophins are inversely related. The demonstration of sex hormone receptors in the pineal gland and melatonin receptors in the reproductive organs is evidence of a complex relationship between melatonin, the hypothalamus, the pituitary, the pineal and the gonads during pubertal growth [98,99].

Gonadotrophin-releasing hormone (GRH) is secreted in a pulsatile manner by neurons in the hypothalamus. Activation of GRH receptors in the pituitary gland controls the release of luteinizing hormone and follicle-stimulating hormone and thus gonad activity. Melatonin has an inhibitory effect on the hypothalamic-pituitary-gonad axis by down-regulating gonodatrophin-releasing hormone gene expression [97,100]. Serum melatonin levels are high during childhood but subsequently decline below a threshold value, signalling the hypothalamus to secrete gonodatrophin-releasing hormone, triggering the onset of puberty [101]. The action of melatonin on the gonads is an indirect effect as pubertal growth and maturation occurs through the action of the sex hormones on other receptors. The inhibitory effect on growth hormone signalling is an effective means of preventing precocious puberty.

Experimentally, it has been demonstrated that melatonin may act directly on the pituitary Gland, inducing growth hormone (GH) and prolactin (PRL) release [17,102,103]. On the other hand, melatonin has been shown to act indirectly on suprachiasmatic nucleus neurons through its receptor inducing the expression of Growth Hormone-Releasing Peptide and related peptides, thus stimulating GH and PRL release from the pituitary [104]. This difference may be species specific.

High levels of melatonin have been found in women with amenorrhoea and in delayed onset of puberty, while low levels have been reported in precocious puberty [105,106]. However, the incidence of scoliosis in precocious puberty appears to be no different from the general population. Human models of endocrine-related disturbances of growth and maturation with a significantly high incidence of scoliosis are limited. There are some notable clinical syndromes with growth disturbance and precocious or delayed puberty, which may provide some insight into the hypothalamic-pituitary-gonad axis.

Prader-Willi syndrome is a genetic hypothalamic-hypophyseal disorder in which growth hormone secretion us usually decreased. Puberty is usually delayed. Up to 80% of Prader-Willi subjects develop scoliosis. Whether there is a corresponding over-secretion of melatonin causing suppression of growth hormone secretion is unknown. The prevalence and magnitude of the scoliosis is not influenced by growth hormone treatment [107]. Likewise, the frequency and severity of the scoliosis in Turner's syndrome (short-statured children), which has 28% prevalence of scoliosis, is not affected by growth hormone therapy [108,109]. Growth hormone does not appear to be a promoter or agent of modification of scoliosis. Recent research suggests that polymorphism at the promoter region of calmodulin-1 gene and the homozygous genotype of growth hormone receptor gene may be associated with high susceptibility to AIS [110]. Scoliosis, sleep disorders and precocious puberty are commonly observed in female patients with Rett syndrome. Three quarters of Rett syndrome patients develop scoliosis by the age of 13 years [111-113]. Studies of children with Rett syndrome showed that the peak secretion of melatonin was normal, but the peak value was at a lower limit for normal children [114,115]. Although scoliosis in Rett syndrome has long been considered neurogenic in type [116], the findings may indicate an underlying melatonin deficiency associated with a high incidence of scoliosis in a genetic condition that affects females.

McCune-Albright syndrome and Jaffe-Lichtenstein syndrome are genetic conditions associated with precocious puberty and endocrine changes, with a high frequency of scoliosis. In a study of patients with polyostotic fibrous dysplasia, the estimated prevalence of scoliosis was 40 to 52% [117]. Half the patients had precocious puberty with no relationship to the presence of scoliosis. The scoliosis was possibly related to the presence of spinal lesions and pelvic obliquity, and biochemically to phosphaturia and hyperparathyroidism, rather than a specific endocrine disorder. Although a neuroendocrine-related association with scoliosis was not evident in this study, a possible melatonin deficiency has been postulated as a potential association in fibrous dysplasia-like disorders by virtue of the failure of melatonin to bind to its RZR/ROR receptors, resulting in changes in the levels of activity of nuclear cAMP that lead to alteration of expression of bone sialoprotein [118].

Scoliosis and precocious or late puberty are common in Neurofibromatosis Type 1. The prevalence of scoliosis is 10 to 20%, with the majority evident before the age of seven years [119,120]. Precocious puberty is usually associated with an optic pathway glioma (OPG). Of the 5% to 25% of NF1 patients who have an OPG [121], up to 39% have precocious puberty [122]. Biochemical analysis of hormones secreted by the pituitary have demonstrated numerous hormonal irregularities [122-125]. Although there has been no research into the possible association of these hormone irregularities and melatonin, is has been postulated that melatonin deficiency, increased serotonin level with disturbed melatonin-serotonin interactions and calmodulin antagonism could be responsible for progression of spinal deformities in neurofibromatosis 1 [126,127].

Lesions of the hypothalamus are frequently associated with precocious puberty, including gliomas, hamartomas, and arachnoid cysts [128,129]. A number of hormonal abnormalities arising from the hypothalamic-pituitary axis have been reported. The studies have concentrated on the pituitary hormones with a systemic effect rather than what effect the tumor may have on melatonin secretion and whether altered melatonin secretion might be related to any systemic hormonal change. Hamartomas may induce precocious puberty either by having gonadotrophin-releasing hormone (GRH) activity or interfere with the antagonists of the normal hypothalamic GRH pulse generator. Melatonin has this potential as a GRH antagonist. Low levels of melatonin have been reported in a case of hypothalamic hamartoma with precocious puberty [34].

The is currently no evidence that genes regulating the synthesis of growth hormone or the gonadotrophins predispose to or modify the development of adolescent idiopathic scoliosis. Although melatonin appears to have an inhibitory role on the gonadotrophin-releasing hormone generator in the hypothalamus, its role as a primary factor or a secondary effect in precocious or delayed puberty and associated scoliosis is unproven. Hormone regulation in growth and maturation and its effect of the development of scoliosis is clearly complex. Future studies of hormonal changes in precocious puberty should include analysis of melatonin levels.

Melatonin, Osteoblasts and Osteoporosis

Melatonin may have a direct effect on osteoblasts and osteoclasts in experimental animals [130,131]. Melatonin has been shown to stimulate the differentiation of both human and animal osteoblasts in cell culture in a dose-dependent manner with a demonstrable increase in procollagen production [132,133]. Its effect on bone homeostasis is due in part to promotion of bone synthesis and in part to down regulation of (receptor activator of nuclear factor KB) RANK-mediated osteoclastic bone resorption [134]. Both melatonin and estrogen retard bone resorption following ovariectomy in experimental animals [135]. The effect of estrogen was augmented by the addition of melatonin in preventing bone resorption [130]. Significantly lower bone mineral densities and lower numbers of osteocytes have been reported in the vertebrae of pinealectomized chickens, almost all of which developed scoliosis, compared with a control group of pineal-intact chickens [136]. The number of osteoblasts was similar in both groups. Experimentally, an association between the pineal deficiency, melatonin deficiency, reduced osteoblast differentiation, reduced bone density and scoliosis has been demonstrated.

Low Bone Mineral Density is a generalized phenomenon in adolescent idiopathic scoliosis [137-140]. The prevalence of adolescent idiopathic scoliosis with osteoporosis is approximately 20 to 38% [141]. Follow-up studies indicated that osteopenia in patients with adolescent idiopathic scoliosis persists [139,142]. No correlation was noted between the severity of the deformity and the bone density [143]. Melatonin and estrogens play a role in the normal vertebral remodelling during the pubertal growth period.

Osteoblast differentiation is probably mediated by melatonin activation of MT2 melatonin receptors. Melatonin is known to inhibit the accumulation of induced cAMP in normal cells due to the coupling of melatonin receptors to an inhibitory protein [144,145]. Normal osteoblasts in cell culture show a dose-dependent decrease in cAMP cell levels with increasing concentrations of melatonin. The response of osteoblasts from idiopathic scoliosis is different, the effect ranging from an increased production of cAMP to a low-grade proportional reduction in cAMP [80]. Because accumulation of high levels of cAMP suppresses osteoblastic function, these findings suggest that melatonin signaling is impaired in osteoblasts isolated from idiopathic scoliosis patients. Such a defect may result in deregulation of osteoblast differentiation and reduced bone density. Whether the resultant osteoporosis is a primary cause of the scoliosis or a secondary effect has not been determined.

Idiopathic Scoliosis and Brain Dysfunction/Lesions

MRIs of the brain and spinal cord can help in the investigation of abnormalities of proprioception, postural equilibrium control, oculo-vestibular function, and vibratory sensation for the purpose of clinical neuromotor assessment of children with idiopathic scoliosis [146-150]. Younger children with progressive idiopathic scoliotic curves with and without neuromotor signs are more likely to have brain stem abnormalities such as Arnold-Chiari type-1 malformation, syringomyelia, or cerebellar tonsillar ectopia [151-156]. However, lesions involving the suprasellar region and pineal gland in juveniles and adolescents have not been implicated in the etiology of idiopathic scoliosis [157].

Conclusion

Although the pineal gland, and in particular melatonin, have been observed to play a major role in the development of scoliosis in experimental animal models, melatonin has no clear role in the etiology of idiopathic scoliosis in humans. The etiology of idiopathic scoliosis remains obscure but is clearly more complex than animal models. Its causal factors and progression are likely to be multifactorial, possibly including genetically predisposed growth receptors susceptible to plasma levels of and/or a balance between the various hormones, involved in pubertal growth, including melatonin. Alteration in melatonin levels due to hypothalamic or pineal pathologies or possible genetic syndromes do not appear to increase the incidence of idiopathic scoliosis. In humans, the role of melatonin and the pineal gland may be permissive, rather than an apparently more direct influence, observed in the animal model. Even then, scoliosis only develops in the majority of experimental animals suggesting that other factors, including genetic susceptibility, may also influence the development of their spine/spinal deformities.

References

[1] Lerner AB, Case JD, Takahashi Y, Lee TH, Mori N: Isolation of melatonin, pineal factor that lightens melanocytes. *J. Am. Chem. Soc.* 1958;80: 2587-2592.

[2] Lerner AB, Case JD, Heinzelmann RV: Structure of melatonin. *J. Am. Chem. Soc.* 1959;81: 6084–6085.

[3] Axelrod J: The pineal gland: a neurochemical transducer. *Science* 1974; 1184: 1341–1348.

[4] Thillard MJ: Deformation de la colonna vertebrale consecutives a lepiphysectomie chez le poussin. *Extrait des Comptes Rendus de l'Association des Anatomistes. XLVI,* 1959:22–26.

[5] Dubousset J, Queneau P, Thillard MJ: Experimental scoliosis induced by pineal and diencephalic lesions in young chickens: its relation with clinical findings in idiopathic scoliosis. *Orthop. Trans.* 1983;7:7.

[6] Machida M, Dubousset J, Satoh T, Murai I, Wood KB, Yamada T, Ryu J: Pathologic mechanism of experimental scoliosis in pinealectomized chickens. *Spine* 2001; 26: E385–391.

[7] Inoh H, Kawakami N, Matsuyama Y, Aoki T, Kanemura T, Natsume N, Iwata H: Correlation between the age of pinealectomy and the development of scoliosis in chickens. *Spine* 2001;26:1014–1021.

[8] Illes T, Horvath G: Pinealectomy and scoliosis. *J. Bone Joint Surg. Am.* 2000;82:1197–1198.

[9] Beuerlein M, Wilson J, Moreau M, Raso VJ, Mahood J, Wang X, Greenhill B, Bagnall KM: The critical stage of pinealectomy surgery after which scoliosis is produced in young chickens. *Spine* 2001; 26: 237–240.

[10] Beuerlein M, Wang X, Moreau M, Raso J, Mahood J, Bagnall K: Development of scoliosis following pinealectomy in young chickens is not the result of an artifact of the surgical procedure. *Microsc. Res. Tech.* 2001; 53: 81–86.

[11] Wang X, Jiang H, Raso J, Moreau M, Mahood J, Zhao J, Bagnall K: Characterization of the scoliosis that develops after pinealectomy in the chicken and comparison with adolescent idiopathic scoliosis in humans. *Spine* 1997; 22: 2626–2635.

[12] Machida M, Dubousset J, Imamura Y, Iwaya T, Yamada T, Kimura J: An experimental study in chickens for the pathogenesis of idiopathic scoliosis. *Spine* 1993; 18: 1609–1615.

[13] Coillard C, Rivard CH: Vertebral deformities and scoliosis. *Eur. Spine J.* 1996; 5: 91–100.

[14] Fagan A, Fazzalari N: Pinealectomy and scoliosis in the chicken: morphology and relationship to melatonin levels. *Proceedings Spine Society* Australia, 2004.

[15] Bagnall KM, Beuerlein M, Johnson P, Wilson J, Raso VJ, Moreau M: Pineal transplantation after pinealectomy in young chickens has no effect on the development of scoliosis. *Spine* 2001; 26: 1022–1027.

[16] Turgut M, Yenisey C, Uysal A, Bozkurt M, Yurtseven ME: The effects of pineal gland transplantation on the production of spinal deformity and serum melatonin level following pinealectomy in the chicken. *Eur. Spine J.* 2003; 12: 487–494.

[17] Zeman M, Buyse J, Lamosova D, Herichova I, Decuypere E: Role of melatonin in the control of growth and growth hormone secretion in poultry. *Domest. Anim. Endocrinol.* 1999; 17: 199–207.

[18] Machida M, Dubousset J, Imamura Y, Iwaya T, Yamada T, Kimura J: Role of melatonin deficiency in the development of scoliosis in pinealectomised chickens. *J. Bone Joint Surg. Br.* 1995; 77: 134–138.

[19] Wang X, Moreau M, Raso VJ, Zhao J, Jiang H, Mahood J, Bagnall K: Changes in serum melatonin levels in response to pinealectomy in the chicken and its correlation with development of scoliosis. *Spine* 1998; 23: 2377–2382.

[20] Nette F, Dolynchuk K, Wang X, Daniel A, Demianczuk C, Moreau M, Raso J, Mahood J, Bagnall K: The effects of exposure to intense, 24 h light on the development of scoliosis in young chickens. *Stud. Health Technol. Inform.* 2002; 91: 1–6.

[21] Cheung KM, Lu DS, Poon AM, Wang T, Luk KD, Leong JC: Effect of melatonin suppression on scoliosis development in chickens by either constant light or surgical pinealectomy. *Spine* 2003; 28: 1941–1944.

[22] Bagnall K, Raso VJ, Moreau M, Mahood J, Wang X, Zhao J: The effects of melatonin therapy on the development of scoliosis after pinealectomy in the chicken. *J. Bone Joint Surg. Am.* 1999; 81: 191–199.

[23] Machida M, Miyashita Y, Murai I, Dubousset J, Yamada T, Kimura J: Role of serotonin for scoliotic deformity in pinealectomized chicken. *Spine* 1997; 22: 1297–1301.

[24] Poon A, Cheung K, Lu D, Leong JC: Changes in melatonin receptors in relation to the development of scoliosis in pinealectomized chickens. *Spine* 2006; 31: 2043-2047.

[25] O'Kelly C, Wang X, Raso J, Moreau M, Mahood J, Zhao J, Bagnall K: The production of scoliosis after pinealectomy in young chickens, rats, and hamsters. *Spine* 1999; 24: 35–43.

[26] Machida M, Murai I, Miyashita Y, Dubousset J, Yamada T, Kimura J: Pathogenesis of idiopathic scoliosis. Experimental study in rats. *Spine* 1999; 24: 1985–1989.

[27] Oyama J, Murai I, Kanazawa K, Machida M: Bipedal ambulation induces experimental scoliosis in C57BL/6J mice with reduced plasma and pineal melatonin levels. *J. Pineal Res.* 2006; 40: 219-224.

[28] Machida M, Dubousset J, Yamada T, Kimura J, Saito M, Shiraishi T, Yamagishi M: Experimental scoliosis in melatonin-deficient C57BL/6J mice without pinealectomy. *J. Pineal Res.* 2006; 41: 1-7.

[29] Cheung KM, Wang T, Poon AM, Carl A, Tranmer B, Hu Y, Luk KD, Leong JC: The effect of pinealectomy on scoliosis development in young nonhuman primates. *Spine* 2005; 30: 2009–13.

[30] Kitay JI: Pineal lesions and precocious puberty: a review. *J. Clin. Endocrinol. Metab.* 1954; 14: 622–625.

[31] Sklar CA, Conte FA, Kaplan SL, Grumbach MM: Human chorionic gonadotropin-secreting pineal tumor: relation to pathogenesis and sex limitation of sexual precocity. *J. Clin. Endocrinol. Metab.* 1981; 53: 656–660.

[32] Rivarola, Belgorosky A, Mendilaharzu H, Vidal G: Precocious puberty in children with tumours of the suprasellar and pineal areas: organic central precocious puberty. *Acta Paediatr.* 2001; 90: 751–756.

[33] Nogueira K, Liberman B, Pimentel-Filho FR, Goldman J, Silva ME, Vieira JO, Buratini JA, Cukiert A: hCG-secreting pineal teratoma

causing precocious puberty: report of two patients and review of the literature. *J. Pediatr. Endocrinol. Metab.* 2002; 15: 1195–1201.

[34] Commentz JC, Helmke K: Precocious puberty and decreased melatonin secretion due to a hypothalamic hamartoma. *Horm. Res.* 1995; 44: 271–275.

[35] Dubousset J: Scoliosis and its pathophysiology: do we understand it? *Spine* 2001; 26: 1001.

[36] Etzioni A, Luboshitzky R, Tiosano D, Ben-Harush M, Goldsher D, Lavie P: Melatonin replacement corrects sleep disturbances in a child with pineal tumor. *Neurology* 1996; 46: 261-263.

[37] Murata J, Sawamura Y, Ikeda J, Hashimoto S, Honma K: Twenty-four hour rhythm of melatonin in patients with a history of pineal and/or hypothalamo-neurohypophyseal germinoma. *J. Pineal Res.* 1998; 25: 159-166.

[38] Day GA, McPhee IB, Tuffley J, Tomlinson F, Chaseling R, Kellie S, Torode I, Sherwood M, Cutbush K, Geddes AJ, Brankoff B: Idiopathic scoliosis and pineal lesions in Australian children. *J. Orthop. Surg.* 2007; 15: 327-333.

[39] Kanemura T, Kawakami N, Deguchi M, Mimatsu K, Iwata H: Natural course of experimental scoliosis in pinealectomized chickens. *Spine* 1997; 22: 1563–1567.

[40] Stokes IA, Aronsson DD: Disc and vertebral wedging in patients with progressive scoliosis. *J. Spinal Disord.* 2001; 14: 317–322.

[41] Parent S, Labelle H, Skalli W, Latimer B, de Guise J: Morphometric analysis of anatomic scoliotic specimens. *Spine* 2002; 27: 2305–2311.

[42] Stokes IA, Spence H, Aronsson DD, Kilmer N: Mechanical modulation of vertebral body growth. Implications for scoliosis progression. *Spine* 1996; 21: 1162–1167.

[43] Mehlman CT, Araghi A, Roy DR: Hyphenated history: the Hueter-Volkmann law. *Am. J. Orthop.* 1997; 26: 798–800.

[44] Somerville EW: Rotational lordosis: the development of the single curve. *J. Bone Joint Surg. Br.* 1952; 34: 421–427.

[45] Dickson RA, Lawton JO, Archer IA, Butt WP: The pathogenesis of idiopathic scoliosis. Biplanar spinal asymmetry. *J. Bone Joint Surg. Br.* 1984; 66: 8–15.

[46] Guo X, Chau WW, Chan YL, Cheng JC: Relative anterior spinal overgrowth in adolescent idiopathic scoliosis. Results of disproportionate endochondral-membranous bone growth. *J. Bone Joint Surg. Br.* 2003; 85: 1026–1031.

[47] Cheung KM, Wang T, Hu YG, Leong JC: Primary thoracolumbar scoliosis in pinealectomized chickens. *Spine* 2003; 28: 2499–2504.

[48] Turhan E, Acaroglu E, Bozkurt G, Alanay A, Yazici M, Surat A: Unilateral enucleation affects the laterality but not the incidence of scoliosis in pinealectomized chicken. *Spine.* 2006; 31: 133-138.

[49] Taylor L: Inheritance of kypho-scoliosis unassociated with other defects in chickens. *Poult. Sci.* 1955; 34: 1225.

[50] Taylor LW: Kyphoscoliosis in a long-term selection experiment with chickens. *Avian. Dis.* 1971; 15: 376–390.

[51] Rucker R, Opsahl W, Abbott U, Greve C, Kenney C, Stern R: Scoliosis in chickens. A model for the inherited form of adolescent scoliosis. *Am. J. Pathol.* 1986; 123: 585–588.

[52] McCarrey JR, Abbott UK, Benson DR, Riggins RS: Genetics of scoliosis in chickens. *J. Hered.* 1981; 72: 6–10.

[53] Riggins RS, Abbott UK, Ashmore CR, Rucker RB, McCarrey JR: Scoliosis in chickens. *J. Bone Joint Surg. Am.* 1977; 59: 1020–1026.

[54] Opsahl W, Abbott U, Kenney C, Rucker R: Scoliosis in chickens: responsiveness of severity and incidence to dietary copper. *Science* 1984; 225: 440–442.

[55] Greve C, Trachtenberg E, Opsahl W, Abbott U, Rucker R: Diet as an external factor in the expression of scoliosis in a line of susceptible chickens. *J. Nutr.* 1987; 117: 189–193.

[56] Turgut M, Yenisey C, Bozkurt M, Ergin F, Bicakci T: Analysis of zinc and magnesium levels in pinealectomized chicks. *Biolog. Trace Element. Res.* 2006; 113: 67-67.

[57] Harrington PR: The etiology of idiopathic scoliosis. *Clin. Orthop. Relat. Res.* 1977; 126: 17–25.

[58] Miller NH: Genetics of familial idiopathic scoliosis. *Clin. Orthop. Relat. Res.* 2002; 401: 60–64.

[59] Riseborough EJ, Wynne-Davies R: A genetic survey of idiopathic scoliosis in Boston, Massachusetts. *J. Bone Joint Surg. Am.* 1973; 55: 974–982.

[60] Carr AJ: Adolescent idiopathic scoliosis in identical twins. *J. Bone Joint Surg. Br.* 1990: 72: 1077.

[61] Kesling KL, Reinker KA: Scoliosis in twins. A meta-analysis of the literature and report of six cases. *Spine* 1997; 22: 2009–2015.

[62] van Rhijn LW, Jansen EJ, Plasmans CM, Veraart BE: Curve characteristics in monozygotic twins with adolescent idiopathic

scoliosis: three new twin pairs and a review of the literature. *Acta Orthop. Scand.* 2001; 72: 621–625.

[63] Wise CA, Barnes R, Gillum J, Herring JA, Bowcock AM, Lovett M: Localization of susceptibility to familial idiopathic scoliosis. *Spine* 2000; 25: 2372–2380.

[64] Chan V, Fong GC, Luk KD, Yip B, Lee MK, Wong MS, Lu DD, Chan TK: A genetic locus for adolescent idiopathic scoliosis linked to chromosome 19p13.3. *Am. J. Hum. Genet.* 2002; 71: 401–406.

[65] Salehi LB, Mangino M, De Serio S, De Cicco D, Capon F, Semprini S, Pizzuti A, Novelli G, Dallapiccola B: Assignment of a locus for autosomal dominant idiopathic scoliosis (IS) to human chromosome 17p11. *Hum. Genet.* 2002; 111: 401–404.

[66] Justice CM, Miller NH, Marosy B, Zhang J, Wilson AF: Familial idiopathic scoliosis: evidence of an X-linked susceptibility locus. *Spine* 2003; 28: 589–594.

[67] Machida M, Dubousset J, Imamura Y, Miyashita Y, Yamada T, Kimura J: Melatonin. A possible role in pathogenesis of adolescent idiopathic scoliosis. *Spine* 1996; 21: 1147–1152.

[68] Sadat-Ali M, al-Habdan I, al-Othman A: Adolescent idiopathic scoliosis. Is low melatonin a cause? *Joint Bone Spine* 2000; 67: 62–64.

[69] Machida M, Dubousset J, Yamada T, Kimura J: Serum melatonin levels in adolescent idiopathic scoliosis prediction and prevention for curve progression – a prospective study. *J. Pineal Res.* 2009; 46: 344-348.

[70] Bagnall KM, Raso VJ, Hill DL, Moreau M, Mahood JK, Jiang H, Russell G, Bering M, Buzzell GR: Melatonin levels in idiopathic scoliosis. Diurnal and nocturnal serum melatonin levels in girls with adolescent idiopathic scoliosis. *Spine* 1996; 21: 1974–1978.

[71] Hilibrand AS, Blakemore LC, Loder RT, Greenfield ML, Farley FA, Hensinger RN, Hariharan M: The role of melatonin in the pathogenesis of adolescent idiopathic scoliosis. *Spine* 1996; 21: 1140–1146.

[72] Fagan AB, Kennaway DJ, Sutherland AD: Total 24-hour melatonin secretion in adolescent idiopathic scoliosis. A case-control study. *Spine* 1998; 23: 41–46.

[73] Brodner W, Krepler P, Nicolakis M, Langer M, Kaider A, Lack W, Waldhauser F: Melatonin and adolescent idiopathic scoliosis. *J. Bone Joint Surg. Br.* 2000; 82: 399–403.

[74] Dubousset J: Point of view. *Spine* 1996; 21: 1978.

[75] Suh K, Lee S, Kim S, Kim Y, Lee J: Pineal gland metabolism in patients with adolescent idiopathic scoliosis. *J. Bone Joint Surg.* 2007; 89: 66-71.

[76] Sobajima S, Kin A, Baba I, Kanbara K, Semoto Y, Abe M: Implication for melatonin and its receptor in the spinal deformities of hereditary lordoscoliotic rabbits. *Spine* 2003; 28: 554–558.

[77] Morcuende JA, Minhas R, Dolan L, Stevens J, Beck J, Wang K, Weinstein SL, Sheffield V: Allelic variants of human melatonin 1A receptor in patients with familial adolescent idiopathic scoliosis. *Spine* 2003; 28: 2025–2029.

[78] Qiu X, Tang N, Yeung H, Cheng J, Qiu Y: Lack of association between the promoter polymorphism of the MTNR1A gene and adolescent idiopathic scoliosis. *Spine* 2008; 33: 2204-2207.

[79] Qiu X, Tang N, Yeung H, Lee K, Hung V, Ng B, Ma S, Kwok R, Qin L, Qiu Y, Cheng J: Melatonin receptor 1B (MTNR1B) gene polymorphism is associated with the occurrence of adolescent idiopathic scoliosis. *Spine* 2007; 32: 1748-1753.

[80] Moreau A, Wang DS, Forget S, Azeddine B, Angeloni D, Fraschini F, Labelle H, Poitras B, Rivard CH, Grimard G: Melatonin signaling dysfunction in adolescent idiopathic scoliosis. *Spine* 2004; 29: 1772–81.

[81] Axelrod J, Weissenbch H: Enzymatic O-methylation of N-acetylserotonin to melatonin. *Science* 1960; 131: 312-1315.

[82] Day G, Szvetko A, Griffiths L, McPhee IB, Tuffley T, Labrom R, Askin G, Woodland P, McClosky E, Torode I, Tomlinson F: Low expression of the ASMT gene in idiopathic and congenital scoliosis vertebral growth plates (unpublished).

[83] Wang H, Wu Z, Zhuang Q, Fei Q, Zhang J, Liu Y, Wang Y, Ding Y, Qiu G: Association study of tryptophan hydroxylase 1 and arylalkylamine N-acetyltransferase polymorphisms with adolescent idiopathic scoliosis in Han Chinese. *Spine* 2008; 33: 2199-2203.

[84] Pozo D, Reiter R, Calvo J, Guerrero J: Inhibition of cerebellar nitric oxide synthase and cyclic GMP production by melatonin via complex formation with calmodulin. *J. Cell Biochem.* 1997; 65: 430-442.

[85] Akel I, Demirkiran G, Alanay A, Karahan S, Marcucio R, Acaroglu E: The effect of calmodulin antagonists on scoliosis: bipedal C57BL/6 mice model. *Eur. Spine J.* 2009; 18: 499-505.

[86] Akel I, Kocak O, Bozkurt G, Alanay A, Marcucio R, Acaroglu E: The effect of calmodulin antagonists on experimental scoliosis: a pinealectomized chicken model. *Spine*;2009; 34: 533-539.

[87] Kindsfater K, Lowe T, Lawellin D, Weinstein D, Akmakjian J: Levels of platelet calmodulin for the prediction of progression and severity of adolescent idiopathic scoliosis. *J. Bone Joint Surg. Am.* 1994; 76:

1186–1192.
[88] Lowe T, Lawellin D, Smith D, Price C, Haher T, Merola A, O'Brien M: Platelet calmodulin levels in adolescent idiopathic scoliosis: do the levels correlate with curve progression and severity? *Spine* 2002; 27: 768–775.
[89] Qiu G, Li J, Liu Y, Wu Z, Zhao Z: Expression of calmodulin in the articular process of vertebrae of adolescent idiopathic scoliosis patients. *Zhonghua Yi Xue Za Zhi* 2006; 86: 2017-2020.
[90] Zhao Y, Qiu G: Expression of calmodulin and nNOS in the paraspinal muscles in idiopathic scoliosis. *Zhonghua Yi Xue Za Zhi* 2004; 84: 1358-1361.
[91] Meyer S, More R, Yarom R: Platelet pathology in minimal curve idiopathic scoliosis: an attempt to predict curve progression. *J. Orthop. Res.* 1987; 5: 330-336.
[92] Liebergall M, Floman Y, Eldor A: Functional, biochemical and structural anomalies in platelets of patients with idiopathic scoliosis. *J. Spinal. Disord.* 1989; 2: 126-130.
[93] Kahmann R, Donohue J, Bradford D, White J, Rao G: Platelet function in adolescent idiopathic scoliosis. *Spine* 1992; 17: 145-148.
[94] Lowe TG, Burwell RG, Dangerfield PH: Platelet calmodulin levels in adolescent idiopathic scoliosis (AIS): can they predict curve progression and severity? Summary of an electronic focus group debate of the IBSE. *Eur. Spine J.* 2004; 13: 257–265.
[95] Glass JD, Knotts LK: A brain site for the antigonadal action of melatonin in the white-footed mouse (Peromyscus leucopus): involvement of the immunoreactive GnRH neuronal system. *Neuroendocrinology* 1987; 46: 48–55.
[96] Kennaway DJ, Rowe SA: Melatonin binding sites and their role in seasonal reproduction. *J. Reprod. Fertil.* 1995;Suppl. 49: 423–435.
[97] Roy D, Belsham DD: Melatonin receptor activation regulates GnRH gene expression and secretion in GT1-7 GnRH neurons: Signal transduction mechanisms. *J. Biol. Chem.* 2001; 277: 251–258.
[98] Luboshitzky R, Dharan M, Goldman D, Herer P, Hiss Y, Lavie P: Seasonal variation of gonadotropins and gonadal steroids receptors in the human pineal gland. *Brain Res. Bull.* 1997; 44: 665–670.
[99] Sanchez JJ, Abreu P, Gonzalez-Hernandez T, Hernandez A, Prieto L, Alonso R: Estrogen modulation of adrenoceptor responsiveness in the female rat pineal gland: differential expression of intracellular estrogen receptors. *J. Pineal Res.* 2004; 37: 26–35.

[100] Balík A, Kretschmannová K, Mazna P, Svobodová I, Zemková H. Melatonin action in neonatal gonadotrophs. *Physiol. Res.* 2004; 53 (Suppl. 1): S153–S166.

[101] Silman R: Melatonin and the human gonodatrophin-releasing hormone pulse generator. *J. Endocrinol.* 1991; 128: 7-11.

[102] Falcón J, Besseau L, Fazzari D, Attia J, Gaildrat P, Beauchaud M, Boeuf G: Melatonin modulates secretion of growth hormone and prolactin by trout pituitary glands and cells in culture. *Endocrinology* 2003; 144: 4648–4658.

[103] Griffiths D, Bjoro T, Gautvik K, Haug E: Melatonin reduces the production and secretion of prolactin and growth hormone from rat pituitary cells in culture. *Acta Physiol. Scand.* 1987; 131: 43–49.

[104] Chowdhury VS, Yamamoto K, Saeki I, Hasunuma I, Shimura T, Tsutsui K: Melatonin Stimulates the release of growth hormone and prolactin by a possible induction of the expression of frog growth hormone-releasing peptide and its related peptide-2 in the amphibian hypothalamus. *Endocrinology* 2008; 149: 962–970.

[105] Waldhauser F, Weiszenbacher G, Frisch H, Zeitlhuber U, Waldhauser M, Wurtman R: Fall in nocturnal serum melatonin during prepuberty and pubescence. *Lancet* 1984; 1(8373): 362-365.

[106] Waldhauser F, Boepple P, Schemper M, Mansfield M, Crowley W Jr: Serum melatonin in central precocious puberty is lower than in age-matched prepubertal children. *J. Clin. Endocrinol. Metab.* 1991; 73: 793-796.

[107] de Lind van Wijngaarden R, de Klerk L, Festen D, Duivenvoorden H, Otten B, Hokken-Koelega A: Randomized controlled trial to investigate the effects of growth hormone treatment on scoliosis in children with Prader-Willi syndrome. *J. Clin. Endocrinol. Metab.* 2009; 94: 1274-80.

[108] Bolar K, Hoffman A, Maneatis T, Lippe B: Long-term safety of recombinant human growth hormone in turner syndrome. *J. Clin. Endocrinol. Metab.* 2008; 93: 344-351.

[109] Day G, McPhee IB, Batch J, Tomlinson FH: Growth rates and the prevalence and progression of scoliosis in short-statured children on Australian growth hormone treatment programmes. *Scoliosis J.* 2007; 2:3.

[110] Zhuang Q, Wu Z, Qiu G: Is polymorphism of CALM1 gene or growth hormone receptor gene associated with susceptibility to adolescent idiopathic scoliosis? *Zhonghua Yi Xue Za Zhi* 2007; 87: 2198-2202.

[111] Ager S, Fyfe S, Christodoulou J, Jacoby P, Schmidt L, Leonard H: Predictors of scoliosis in Rett syndrome. *J. Child Neurol.* 2006; 21: 809-813.
[112] Huang T, Lubicky J, Hammerberg K : Scoliosis in Rett syndrome. *Orthop. Rev.* 1994; 23: 931-937.
[113] Harrison D, Webb PJ: Scoliosis in the Rett syndrome: natural history and treatment. *Brain Dev.* 1990; 12: 154-156.
[114] Miyamoto A, Oki J, Takahashi S, Okuno A: Serum melatonin kinetics and long-term melatonin treatment for sleep disorders in Rett syndrome. *Brain Dev.* 1999; 21: 59-62.
[115] Yamashita Y, Matsuishi T, Murakami Y, Kato H: Sleep disorder in Rett syndrome and melatonin treatment. *Brain Dev.* 1999; 21: 570.
[116] Lidstrom J, Stokland E, Hagberg B: Scoliosis in Rett syndrome. Clinical and biological aspects. *Spine* 1994; 19: 1632-1635.
[117] Leet AI, Magur E, Lee JS, Wientroub, Robey PG, Collins MT: Fibrous dysplasia in the spine: Prevalence of lesions and association with scoliosis. *J. Bone Joint Surg.* 2004; 86A: 531-537.
[118] Abdel-Wanis M, Tsuchiya H: Melatonin deficiency and fibrous dysplasia: might a relation exist? *Med. Hypotheses* 2002; 59: 552-554.
[119] Crawford AH, Herrera-Soto J: Scoliosis associated with neurofibromatosis. *Orthop. Clin. North America* 2007; 38(4): 553-562.
[120] Durrani A, Crawford AH, Chouhdry S, Saifuddin A, Morley T: Modulation of spinal deformities in patients with neurofibromatosis type 1. *Spine* 2000; 25: 69-75.
[121] Listernick R, Ferner R, Liu G, Gutmann D: Optic pathway gliomas in neurofibromatosis-1: controversies and recommendations. *Annul. Neurol.* 2007; 61: 189-198.
[122] Habiby R, Silverman B, Listernick R, Charrow J: Precocious puberty in children with neurofibromatosis type 1. *J. Pediatr.* 1995; 126: 364-367.
[123] Huguenin M, Trivin C, Zerah M, Doz F, Brugieres L, Brauner R: Adult height after cranial irradiation for optic pathway tumors: relationship with neurofibromatosis. *J. Pediatr.* 2003; 142(6): 699-703.
[124] De Sanctis V, Corrias A, Rizzo V, Bertelloni S, Urso L, Galluzzi F, Pasquino A, Pozzan G, Guarneri M, Cisternino M, De Luca F, Gargantini L, Pilotta A, Sposito M, Tonini G: Etiology of central precocious puberty in males: the results of the Italian Study Group for Physiopathology of Puberty. *J. Pediatr. Endocrin. Metab.* 2000;13 Suppl 1: 687-693.

[125] Collet-Solberg P. Sernyak H, Satin-Smith M, Katz L, Molloy P, Moshang T Jr: Endocrine outcome in long-term survivors of low-grade hypothalamic/chiasmatic glioma. *Clin. Endocrinol.* (Oxf) 1997; 47: 79-85.

[126] Abdel-Wanis M, Kawahara N: Hypophosphatemic osteomalacia in neurofibromatosis 1: hypotheses for pathogenesis and higher incidence of spinal deformity. *Med. Hypotheses* 2002; 59: 183-185.

[127] Abdel-Wanis M, Kawahara N: Aetiology of spinal deformities in neurofibromatosis 1: new hypotheses. *Med. Hypotheses* 2001; 56: 400-404.

[128] Zuniga OF, Tanner S, Wild W, Mosier HD Jr: Hamartoma of CNS associated with precocious puberty. *Am. J. Dis. Child.* 1983; 137: 127-133.

[129] Trivin C, Couto-Silva A, Sainte-Rose C, Chemaitilly W, Kalifa C, Doz F, Zerah M, Brauner R: Presentation and evolution of organic central precocious puberty according to the type of CNS lesion. *Clin Endocrinol.* (Oxf) 2006; 65: 239-245.

[130] Ladizesky M, Boggio V, Albornoz L, Castrillon P, Mautalen C, Cardinali D: Melatonin increases oestradiol-induced bone formation in ovariectomized rats. *J. Pineal Res.* 2003; 34: 143-151.

[131] Cardinali D, Ladizesky M, Boggio V, Cutrera R, Mautalen C: Melatonin effects on bone: experimental facts and clinical perspectives. *J. Pineal Res.* 2003; 34: 81-87.

[132] Roth JA, Kim BG, Lin WL and Cho MI.: Melatonin promotes osteoblast differentiation and bone formation. *J. Biol. Chem.* 1999; 274: 22041–22047.

[133] Nakade O, Koyama H, Ariji H, Yajima A, Kaku T: Melatonin stimulates proliferation and type I collagen synthesis in human bone cells in vitro. *J. Pineal Res.* 1999; 27: 106–110.

[134] Koyama H, Nakade O, Takada Y, Kaku T, Lau KH: Melatonin at pharmacologic doses increases bone mass by suppressing resorption through down-regulation of the RANKL-mediated osteoclast formation and activation. *J. Bone Miner. Res.* 2002; 17: 1219–1229.

[135] Ladizesky MG, Cutrera RA, Boggio V, Somoza J, Centrella JM, Mautalen C, Cardinali DP: Effect of melatonin on bone metabolism in ovariectomized rats. *Life Sci.* 2001; 70: 557–565.

[136] Turgut M, Kaplan S, Turgut AT, Aslan H, Güvenc T, Çullu E, Erdoğan S: Morphological, stereological and radiological changes in

pinealectomized chicken cervical vertebrae. *J. Pineal Res.* 2005; 39: 392–399.
[137] Cook SD, Harding AF, Morgan EL, Nicholson RJ, Thomas KA, Whitecloud TS, Ratner ES. Trabecular bone mineral density in idiopathic scoliosis. *J. Pediatr. Orthop.* 1987; 7: 168-174.
[138] Thomas KA, Cook SD, Skalley TC, Renshaw SV, Makuch RS, Gross M, Whitecloud TS, Bennett JT. Lumbar spine and femoral neck bone mineral density in idiopathic scoliosis: a follow-up study. *J. Pediatr. Orthop.* 1992; 12: 235-240.
[139] Cheng JC, Qin L, Cheung CS, Sher AH, Lee KM, Ng SWE GUO X: Generalized low areal and volumetric bone mineral density in adolescent idiopathic scoliosis. *J. Bone Miner. Res.* 2000; 15: 1587–1595.
[140] Sadat-Ali M, al-Othman A, Bubshait D, al-Dakheel D: Does scoliosis causes low bone mass? A comparative study between siblings. *Eur. Spine J.* 2008; 17: 944-947.
[141] Li XF, Li H, Liu ZD, Dai LY: Low bone mineral status in adolescent idiopathic scoliosis. *Eur. Spine J.* 2008; 17: 1431-1440.
[142] Cheng JC, Guo X, Sher AH: Persistent osteopenia in adolescent idiopathic scoliosis. A longitudinal follow-up study. *Spine* 1999; 24: 1218-1222.
[143] Cheng JC, Tang SP, Guo X, Chan CW, Qin L: Osteopenia in adolescent idiopathic scoliosis: a histomorphometric study. *Spine* (Phila Pa 1976) 2001; 26: E19-23.
[144] Petit L, Lacroix I, de Coppet P, Strosberg AD, Jockers R: Differential signaling of human Mel1a and Mel1b melatonin receptors through the cyclic guanosine 3'-5'-monophosphate pathway. *Biochem. Pharmacol.* 1999; 58: 633–639.
[145] Roka F, Brydon L, Waldhoer M, Strosberg AD, Freissmuth M, Jockers R, Nanoff C: Tight association of the human Mel(1a)-melatonin receptor and G(i): precoupling and constitutive activity. *Mol. Pharmacol.* 1999; 56: 1014–1024.
[146] Gregoric M, Pecak F, Trontelj JV, Dimitrijevic MR: Postural control in scoliosis. A statokinesimetric study in patients with scoliosis due to neuromuscular isorders and in patients with idiopathic scoliosis. *Acta Orthop. Scand.* 1981; 52: 59–63.
[147] Keessen W, Crowe A, Hearn M: Proprioceptive accuracy in idiopathic scoliosis. *Spine* 1992; 17: 149–55.

[148] McInnes E, Hill DL, Raso VJ, Chetner B, Greenhill BJ, Moreau MJ: Vibratory response in adolescents who have idiopathic scoliosis. *J. Bone Joint Surg. Am.* 1991; 73: 1208–1212.

[149] Sahlstrand T, Petruson B: A study of labyrinthine function in patients with adolescent idiopathic scoliosis. I. An electro-nystagmographic study. *Acta Orthop. Scand.* 1979; 50: 759–769.

[150] Yamada K, Yamamoto H, Nakagawa Y, Tezuka A, Tamura T, Kawata S: Etiology of idiopathic scoliosis. *Clin. Orthop. Relat. Res.* 1984; 184: 50–57.

[151] Inoue M, Minami S, Nakata Y, Otsuka Y, Takaso M, Kitahara H, Tokunaga M, Isobe K, Moriya H. Preoperative MRI analysis of patients with idiopathic scoliosis: a prospective study. *Spine* 2005; 30: 108–14.

[152] Morcuende JA, Dolan LA, Vazquez JD, Jirasirakul A, Weinstein SL: A prognostic model for the presence of neurogenic lesions in atypical idiopathic scoliosis. *Spine* 2004; 29: 51–58.

[153] Inoue M, Nakata Y, Minami S, Kitahara H, Otsuka Y, Isobe K, Takaso M, Tokunaga M, Itabashi T, Nishikawa S, Moriya H: Idiopathic scoliosis as a presenting sign of familial neurologic abnormalities. *Spine* 2003; 28: 40–45.

[154] Chartier A, Martinot A, Dhellemmes P, Vallee L, Lamblin MD, Goran C, Leclerc F: Chiari type I malformation in children: presentation in 34 cases [in French]. *Arch. Pediatr.* 2002; 9: 789–796.

[155] Cheng JC, Guo X, Sher AH, Chan YL, Metreweli C: Correlation between curve severity, somatosensory evoked potentials, and magnetic resonance imaging in adolescent idiopathic scoliosis. *Spine* 1999; 24: 1679–1684.

[156] Emery E, Redondo A, Rey A: Syringomyelia and Arnold Chiari in scoliosis initially classified as idiopathic: experience with 25 patients. *Eur. Spine J.* 1997; 6: 158–162.

[157] Pradilla G, Jallo G: Arachnoid cysts: case series and review of the literature. *Neurosurg. Focus* 2007; 22(2): E7.

Index

A

acid, 28, 30
AD, 153, 159
adaptation, 53
adjustment, 62
adolescent idiopathic scoliosis, viii, x, 40, 43, 91, 93, 97, 98, 100, 101, 102, 103, 132, 133, 135, 137, 142, 143, 146, 149, 151, 153, 154, 155, 156, 159, 160
adolescents, 50, 58, 64, 84, 94, 107, 115, 121, 132, 133, 135, 143, 147, 160
adults, 59, 112, 115
adverse event, 90
aetiology, x, 70, 137
age, vii, viii, 1, 6, 9, 10, 17, 31, 35, 36, 40, 58, 64, 74, 79, 81, 82, 84, 85, 86, 87, 92, 93, 94, 95, 107, 125, 140, 144, 145, 148, 156
aging process, 74
amino, 28, 30
amino acid(s), 30
amphibia, 156
androgen(s), 24, 27, 44, 45, 46
angulation, 56, 58, 83, 110
ankles, 125, 126
ANOVA, viii, 74, 79
antagonism, 145
anxiety, 113
apex, 6, 7, 33, 99, 115, 140

applications, 132
arthrodesis, 102
arthrogryposis, 93
arthrogryposis multiplex congenita, 93
assessment, 18, 19, 53, 75, 76, 78, 84, 85, 86, 95, 112, 132, 147
assessment procedures, 84
asymmetry, 34, 83, 92, 93, 108, 109, 122, 151
asymptomatic, 66, 94, 132
athletes, 85
atrophy, 93
authorities, 60
autonomy, 74
autopsy, 3
autosomal dominant, 20, 21, 22, 23, 153
autosomal recessive, 19, 21, 22, 23, 24

B

back pain, 89, 94, 107, 109, 114
backpack carriage, ix, 119, 122, 123, 124, 125, 128, 130, 131
base, 123
bending, 32, 35, 92, 96, 99, 108, 114
binding globulin, 45
biomechanical factors, vii, viii, 49, 58, 91, 93
biomechanics, 84
bipedal, 140, 143, 154

blindness, 141
blood, 24, 25, 26, 96, 99
body composition, 44
body shape, 83
body weight, 122, 124, 126, 127, 128, 129, 139
bone, 8, 24, 28, 35, 38, 39, 40, 41, 44, 45, 46, 71, 85, 87, 93, 94, 99, 100, 145, 146, 151, 158, 159
bone age, 8, 35
bone cells, 158
bone form, 93, 158
bone growth, 28, 151
bone mass, 24, 28, 44, 45, 93, 158, 159
bone resorption, 93, 146
boys, 134
brain, 139, 147, 155
brain stem, 147
Brazil, vii, viii, 73, 74, 75, 76, 77, 82, 86
breathing, 62, 63, 123
bruxism, 57

C

calcium, 100, 142
calibration, 89
candidates, 21, 97
carbon, 34, 120
carbon dioxide, 34, 120
carcinogenicity, 95, 99
cardiovascular disease, 18
cardiovascular function, 138
cardiovascular system, 120
cartilage, 9
case study, ix, 105, 110, 113
casting, 97
Caucasian population, 93
cell biology, 87
cell culture, 146, 147
cellular calcium, 142
Census, 88
central nervous system (CNS), 93
cerebral palsy, 93
challenges, 100
Chicago, 4

chicken, ix, 137, 140, 141, 143, 149, 150, 152, 154, 159
childhood, vii, 1, 10, 143
Chile, 90
China, 119
chorionic gonadotropin, 150
chromosome, 20, 21, 43, 142, 153
circadian rhythm, 138, 139
citizens, 75
clarity, 95
classes, 6
classification, vii, 10, 80, 83, 98, 102
claustrophobia, 114
clinical diagnosis, viii, 74
clinical examination, 88
clinical syndrome, 144
CNS, 93, 158
cobalt, 99
coding, 2, 26
collaboration, 65
collagen, viii, 91, 158
communication, 19, 20
community, 52, 87
compatibility, 22, 23
complexity, 41, 63
compliance, 38, 98
complications, viii, 83, 91, 97
composition, 76
compression, 3, 40
computer, 88, 89
concordance, 21, 142
Congress, 89
connective tissue, 94
Consensus, 67
consent, 76
construction, 83
contracture, 38
control, ix, 119, 121, 128, 130, 132, 133
control group, 60, 143, 146
controlled studies, 52, 53
controversial, 113
controversies, 157
cooperation, 20
copper, 141, 152

correlation(s), 50, 54, 55, 56, 57, 61, 64, 66, 67, 69, 83, 93, 146, 149
cortical bone, 27, 45
cosmetic, 34
cost, 52, 75, 88
cotton, 56
counseling, 18, 20, 111
critical period, 24
cross links, 41
cross-sectional study, 67
CT, 19, 151
CT scan, 19
culture, 146, 147, 156
cycles, 125
cyst, 139

dissociation, 30
distribution, 11, 12, 13, 14, 15, 16, 17, 87, 112
diversity, 50
dizygotic, 20
dizziness, 113
DNA, 17, 19, 100
doctors, 10
dominance, 69
dough, 3
down-regulation, 158
draft, 21
duration, 124, 129, 130, 132, 135
dysplasia, 94, 145, 157

D

daily living, 74, 76, 87
data analysis, 125
database, 53
decortication, 38
defects, viii, 17, 34, 55, 65, 91, 93, 94, 152
deficiency, x, 24, 45, 53, 121, 137, 140, 145, 146, 149, 157
deformation, 4, 58, 60, 120
dental restorations, 53
depression, 33
deprivation, 141
depth, viii, 74, 78, 81, 83, 84, 85
deregulation, 147
detectable, 69
detection, 60, 75, 83, 88, 109
deterrence, 98
deviation, 3, 6, 34, 56, 61, 62, 83
diabetes, 18
digestion, 27, 28, 29
disability, 34, 115
disclosure, 76
discs, 39, 74
diseases, 5, 17, 18
dislocation, 5
disorder, 20, 57, 58, 68, 113, 144, 145, 157
displacement, 34, 60
disproportionate growth, 93

E

eczema, 85
edema, 85
editors, 71
education, 63, 115
elderly population, vii, viii, 74, 75, 85, 86, 90
elders, 88
electrical properties, 30
electrodes, 110
elongation, 37
email, 119
e-mail, 1
EMG, 67, 69, 70
encoding, 2
endocrine, 2, 5, 24, 26, 41, 94, 138, 144, 145
endocrine disorders, 5
energy, 122
engineering, 88
environment, 141
environmental factors, 18
enzyme(s), 2, 24, 26, 27, 28, 29, 142
epidemic, 59
epidemiologic, 75, 76
epidemiologic studies, 75
epiphysis, 8, 10
equality, 43

equilibrium, 51, 53, 62, 85, 121, 123, 130, 132, 147
equipment, 78, 84
estrogen, 2, 24, 31, 41, 44, 45, 46, 146, 155
etiology, vii, ix, x, 5, 42, 49, 53, 58, 61, 92, 119, 137, 139, 147, 152
evidence, ix, 20, 21, 43, 50, 52, 53, 54, 55, 60, 62, 64, 65, 66, 68, 70, 86, 110, 120, 131, 143, 146, 153
evoked potential, 95, 160
evolution, 158
examinations, 10, 17, 19, 50, 57, 58, 59, 62, 64
excision, 3, 39, 96
exclusion, 54
excretion, 142
exercise, 35, 37, 99, 108, 109, 111
exercise programs, 109
exons, 2, 28
experimental pinealectomy, ix, 137, 138, 140, 143
expertise, 109
exposure, 27, 149
extensor, 112, 124

F

facial asymmetry, 50, 61, 62, 64
families, 20, 21, 59, 64, 107
family history, 18, 93
family members, 19
fatigue, 124, 134
female rat, 155
fibrous dysplasia, 145, 157
films, 10, 35, 95, 98, 99
financial, 59
fixation, 4, 40, 95, 98, 99
flank, 31
flaws, 53
flexibility, 4, 34, 35, 99, 120
follicle, 143
force, 4, 36, 38, 40, 56, 57, 68, 70, 110, 121, 122, 124, 125, 126, 133
formation, 5, 60, 94, 154, 158
fractures, 45, 74, 85

France, 4, 38, 65, 95, 138
frozen shoulder, 110, 113
fusion, 3, 5, 8, 9, 38, 39, 92, 95, 96, 97, 98, 99, 101, 103, 133

G

gait, ix, 119, 120, 121, 122, 124, 125, 126, 129, 130, 131, 133, 134, 135
gender differences, viii, 74, 79, 83
gene expression, 143, 155
general anaesthesia, 97
generation, 129
genes, 18, 21, 93, 94, 141, 146
genetic defect, 19
genetic disease, 18, 19, 20
genetic information, 19
genetic linkage, 45
genetic marker, 93
genetic syndromes, 148
genetic testing, 18, 19
genetic traits, 2
genetics, vii, 19, 20, 49, 58
genotype, 2, 144
girls, 124, 125, 126, 127, 128, 129, 130, 135
gland, x, 137, 138, 139, 140, 142, 143, 147, 148, 149, 153, 155
glioma, 145, 158
gonads, 143, 144
grades, 7
gravitational potential energy, 122
gravity, 84, 93, 121, 123, 124
growth, vii, 9, 28, 35, 36, 37, 45, 46, 49, 50, 56, 57, 58, 59, 60, 65, 68, 69, 92, 93, 95, 96, 97, 100, 102, 107, 108, 111, 141, 142, 143, 144, 146, 148, 149, 151, 154, 156
growth arrest, 92, 96
growth factor, 93
growth hormone, 93, 144, 146, 149, 156
growth rate, 107
growth spurt, 95
guidelines, 83

H

hair, 31, 85
harmony, 61
Hawaii, 65
health, viii, 50, 52, 59, 61, 62, 63, 65, 75, 76, 85, 88, 115, 116
health care, 52, 61, 65, 88
health promotion, 75
health status, 62
height, 31, 55, 60, 79, 84, 115, 157
hip, 122, 125, 126, 129, 130
hip joint, 129, 130
histogram, 79
history, vii, 35, 98, 102, 112, 114, 132, 151, 157
homeostasis, 28, 31, 146
Hong Kong, 119
hormone(s), x, 24, 100, 137, 138, 139, 143, 144, 145, 146, 148, 149, 156
host, 59
House, 70
housing, 76
human, vii, viii, ix, 1, 10, 21, 24, 30, 43, 45, 46, 66, 67, 74, 88, 89, 103, 137, 138, 140, 141, 142, 146, 153, 154, 155, 156, 158, 159
human body, viii, 74
human genome, 21
human subjects, 66, 67
humidity, 98
hybrid, 98
hyoid, 71
hyperparathyroidism, 145
hypogonadism, 44
hypothalamus, 143, 145, 146, 156
hypothesis, 2, 55, 56, 67, 115

I

iatrogenic, 40, 60
Iceland, 75
ideal, 85
identical twins, 43, 152
identification, 89
iliac crest, 8, 9, 31, 32, 34
ilium, 8
image analysis, 83
image(s), 78, 83, 84, 86, 88, 89, 95, 115, 139
imitation, 150
immobilization, 38
impairments, 109, 120
implants, 96
improvements, ix, 99, 105, 113
impulses, 56
in utero, 5
in vitro, 158
in vivo, 67
incidence, 10, 17, 20, 42, 60, 84, 94, 112, 132, 140, 141, 142, 143, 144, 145, 148, 152, 158
incisors, 60
income, 76
indirect effect, 144
individuals, ix, 2, 20, 21, 22, 23, 38, 69, 81, 83, 85, 86, 90, 92, 97, 105
induction, 156
inequality, 4, 10, 56, 69
infants, 61, 68
infection, 5
informed consent, 19, 52
inheritance, 2, 19, 20, 21, 22, 23, 141
inhibition, 93
injections, 139, 140
injury, 109
inner ear, 51
insertion, 3
interaction, 124, 127, 129, 130
interference, 63
internal fixation, 47
interrelations, 58
intervention, ix, 87, 92, 94, 100, 105, 106, 110, 112, 114, 115, 117
irradiation, 157
IS phenotype, vii, 1, 2, 10, 20, 24, 25, 26, 31, 41
Italy, 1, 2

J

Japan, 75
joint destruction, 38
joints, 51, 125, 126, 130
justification, 56
juveniles, 147

K

kinetics, 125, 126, 135, 157
knees, 32, 108
kyphosis, viii, 4, 10, 40, 74, 83, 84, 85, 87, 90, 113, 123

L

lack of control, 143
laterality, 12, 13, 141, 152
lead, 62, 75, 85, 124, 141, 145
legend, 6
leptin, 93
lesions, x, 93, 137, 145, 147, 148, 150, 151, 157, 160
leucine, 21
life expectancy, 34, 75
life satisfaction, 87
ligand, 2, 30, 31
light, 18, 88, 89, 139, 149, 150
localization, 54
loci, 2, 21, 101
locus, 20, 43, 153
longitudinal study, 102
lordosis, 4, 40, 55, 56, 67, 101, 107, 141, 151
lumbar spine, 4, 106, 108, 141
lung function, 102, 132, 135
luteinizing hormone, 143
lying, 61, 111

M

magnesium, 152

magnetic resonance, 96, 141, 160
magnetic resonance imaging, 96, 141, 160
magnitude, 6, 7, 34, 35, 98, 108, 122, 134, 141, 143, 144
majority, 26, 98, 107, 110, 115, 145, 148
malocclusion, 50, 61, 62, 64, 65, 67
man, 45
management, 42, 47, 95, 98, 99
mandible, 54, 56, 67
manganese, 141
manipulation, 106, 109, 111
mapping, 21
mass, 24, 78, 79, 84, 93, 121, 158, 159
masseter, 69
matter, 23, 52, 61, 85
measurement(s), 7, 33, 83, 84, 88, 89, 90, 109, 111, 112, 113, 114, 125, 131, 133, 135, 142
measures, ix, 120, 134
median, 36
mediation, 56
medical, 3, 19, 20, 52, 59, 100, 114
medication, 114
medicine, 70, 87
melanin, 93
melatonin, vii, x, 100, 137, 138, 139, 140, 142, 143, 144, 145, 146, 147, 148, 149, 150, 151, 153, 154, 155, 156, 157, 158, 159
memory, 92
menstruation, 58
meta-analysis, 43, 152
metabolic disturbances, vii, 49, 58
metabolism, 24, 41, 142, 153, 158
methylation, 154
mice, 27, 44, 45, 46, 140, 150, 154
mineralization, 24
models, x, 22, 23, 24, 137, 140, 143, 144, 147
modifications, 98
monozygotic twins, 20, 152
morphogenesis, 51
morphology, 55, 67, 68, 70, 149
motion, 121, 122, 125, 126, 128, 129, 130
motor control, 121

Index

movement, 121, 134
MR, 159
MRI, 96, 97, 108, 160
MTI, 125
muscle strength, 44, 87
muscles, 21, 51, 57, 69, 110, 121, 122, 130, 143, 155
muscular dystrophy, 93
musculoskeletal, 74, 124
musculoskeletal system, 74
mutation(s), 31, 45, 46
myelodysplasia, 95
myelomeningocele, 5

N

nerve, 94
nervous system, 93, 100
neural network, 88
neurological disorders, vii, 49, 58
neurological disturbances, vii, 49, 58
neuromotor, 147
neurons, 143, 144, 155
neuropathic pain, 94
New Zealand, 110
nitric oxide, 154
nitric oxide synthase, 154
NMR, 66
non-polar, 30
normal children, ix, 119, 131, 144
normal curve, 107
North America, 157
nucleus, 144
numerical analysis, 89

O

obstruction, 132
occlusion, vii, viii, 49, 50, 51, 52, 53, 54, 55, 56, 57, 58, 59, 61, 64, 65, 66, 67, 69, 70
omission, 54
oral cavity, 53, 57
order, 123

organism, 63
organs, 59, 63, 143
orthodontic treatment, viii, 49, 50, 53, 59, 69, 70
orthopedic surgeon, 109
oscillation, 67
ossification, 8, 9
osteoarthritis, 31
osteomalacia, 94, 158
osteoporosis, 40, 44, 74, 85, 87, 146
outpatients, 102
ovariectomy, 146
overweight, ix, 119
oxygen, 34, 120

P

pain, viii, 31, 53, 54, 55, 66, 68, 71, 91, 94, 107, 109, 110, 112, 113, 114, 115, 135
parallel, 6, 59, 85
parameters, 124, 127, 129, 131, 133, 134
parents, 19, 38, 98
participants, 54, 56, 63, 83, 122, 124, 125, 128
pathogenesis, vii, 1, 3, 10, 141, 149, 150, 151, 153, 158
pathology, vii, 1, 10, 96, 113, 143, 155
pathophysiology, 151
pathways, 45
patient age, vii, 1, 10
PCR, 93
pediatrician, 108, 109
pedigree, 18, 19
pelvis, 4, 32, 95, 96, 125, 128
penetrance, 141
peptide(s), 144, 156
percentile, 81, 85
performance, ix, 119, 120, 121, 123, 124, 131
permit, 80, 83
phenotype, vii, 1, 2, 10, 20, 24, 25, 26, 31, 41
Philadelphia, 71, 101
photographs, 19, 80
physical exercise, 35, 36

physical health, 85
physical therapist, 110
physical therapy, vii, 38, 106, 109, 110, 111
physicians, 113
physics, 88
physiology, 85, 138
pilot study, 66, 67
pineal gland, vii, x, 137, 138, 139, 140, 142, 143, 147, 148, 149, 155
pituitary gland, 143, 156
plasma levels, 148
platelets, 143, 155
platform, 55, 56, 121, 125
PM, 90
point mutation, 26, 28, 31
polar, 30
polymorphism(s), 2, 26, 44, 45, 142, 144, 154, 156
polyostotic fibrous dysplasia, 145
poor, 122
population, vii, viii, 1, 2, 10, 18, 20, 24, 26, 28, 75, 85, 86, 87, 91, 95, 107, 109, 113, 144
position effect, 67, 69
postural control, 56, 60, 67, 128
posture, ix, 119, 122, 123, 124, 125, 128, 130, 133, 134, 135
poultry, 139, 149
power, 129, 130
power generation, 129
Prader-Willi syndrome, 144, 156
precocious puberty, 140, 144, 145, 146, 150, 151, 156, 157, 158
predictability, 100
pregnancy, 114
pressure, 121
prevention, 75, 92, 97, 100, 153
primary school, 122, 134
primary teeth, 71
primate, ix, 137
principles, 38, 71
probability, 19, 124
proband(s), 18, 19, 20
professionals, 20, 75, 76
progesterone, 2, 24, 25, 26

prognosis, 9, 101
prolactin, 144, 156
proliferation, 158
promoter, 144, 154
propagation, 88
prophylaxis, 37
protection, 3
proteins, 30, 99
psychiatric disorders, 138
puberty, vii, 1, 9, 10, 24, 107, 140, 144, 145, 146, 150, 151, 156, 157, 158
public health, 88
pulmonary function, ix, 35, 101, 119, 120, 122, 124, 127, 130, 131, 132, 135
pulmonary function test, 135

Q

quality of life, 74, 85
Queensland, 137

R

radiation, 75, 95, 101
range, 128
RE, 65, 71
reactions, 117, 133
reality, 63
receptors, 46, 142, 143, 145, 147, 148, 150, 155, 159
recommendations, 70, 157
reconstruction, 19
recurrence, 18
reflexes, 97
rehabilitation, 53, 75, 87, 106, 112, 113
rehabilitation program, 75
relatives, 19, 142
relief, 38
remodelling, 46, 146
repetitions, 114
reproduction, 143, 155
reproductive organs, 143
requirements, 4, 99
researchers, 61, 84, 139

resection, 96
resistance, 115
resolution, 10
respect, 121
respiration, 130
respiratory, 120, 122, 132, 134
response, 120, 124, 147, 149, 160
responsiveness, 152, 155
restrictions, 37
restrictive lung disease, 34, 94
reticulum, 76
RH, 143, 145
rhythm, 138, 139, 151
risk(s), 18, 19, 40, 52, 57, 59, 61, 62, 85, 95, 96, 98, 107
rodents, 138
rods, 40, 41, 92, 95, 96, 97, 98, 99
roentgen, 3
root, 94

S

sacrum, 31
safety, 156
saturation, 34
scapula, viii, 31, 74, 78, 79, 84, 86, 89
scapular alignment, viii, 74, 82
school, viii, 10, 61, 68, 91, 100, 108, 122, 134, 135
science, 66
scope, 63
secrete, 144
secretin, 150
secretion, x, 137, 142, 144, 145, 149, 151, 153, 155, 156
segregation, 20, 21
self-esteem, 109
self-image, 115
sensation, 147
sensitivity, 54, 112, 133
serotonin, 139, 142, 145, 150
serum, 24, 44, 45, 93, 139, 141, 142, 149, 153, 156
severity, 120, 131

sex, vii, 1, 2, 10, 11, 12, 13, 14, 15, 16, 17, 20, 21, 24, 27, 41, 44, 45, 141, 143, 144, 150
sex hormones, 144
sex steroid, 24, 27, 44, 45
sexuality, 76
Shadow Moiré Technique (SMT), viii, 74, 75
sham, 138
shape, 38
shortness of breath, 31
showing, viii, 2, 23, 24, 25, 26, 91, 115
siblings, 159
side effects, 60
signalling, 142, 143
signs, 19, 61, 107, 147
Singapore, 91
skeleton, 46
skin, 83, 85, 97
sleep disorders, 144, 157
sleep disturbance, 151
social context, 64
social relations, 76
society, 102
software, 76, 78, 79
SP, 87, 159
space, 121
spastic, 94
specialists, 18, 63
species, 144
speech, 63
speed, 122, 124, 129
spinal cord, 50, 62, 64, 94, 101, 108, 139, 147
spinal fusion, 3, 4, 38, 133
splint, 56, 65, 70
spondylolisthesis, 10
Sprague-Dawley rats, 140
Spring, 137
stability, ix, 3, 56, 66, 69, 95, 112, 119, 121, 122, 123, 124, 130, 131, 133, 134
stabilization, 40, 56, 67, 112
standard deviation, viii, 74, 79, 81
standard error, 126, 127, 128, 129
standardization, 84

standardized testing, 86
state(s), 31, 57, 88, 111
statistics, 79
steel, 3
sternocleidomastoid, 67, 69, 70, 71
steroids, 26, 31, 41, 44, 155
stimulation, 106, 109, 110
stress, ix, 20, 24, 63, 85, 119
stretching, 56
structural changes, 24, 34
structural variation, 55
structure, 30, 85
students, 135
subgroups, 9
substitution(s), 30
suppression, 139, 144, 150
suprachiasmatic nucleus, 144
surface area, 85
surgical intervention, 92, 94, 95
survivors, 158
susceptibility, 43, 144, 148, 153, 156
Sweden, 45
symmetry, 122
sympathetic nervous system, 93, 100
symptomology, 62
symptoms, vii, 31, 94, 107, 113
syndrome, 89, 94, 96, 97, 102, 144, 145, 156, 157
synthesis, 138, 142, 146, 158
syringomyelia, 5, 93, 147

T

tamoxifen, 143
target, 2
techniques, 4, 42, 64
technology, 99
teens, 2, 26, 28
teeth, 53, 56, 61
temporomandibular disorders, 66, 68, 69
tendon, 21
tension, 34, 56, 120
testing, 19, 100, 135
testosterone, 2, 24, 26, 44, 45
textbook, 3

Thailand, 87
therapeutic approaches, 50
therapy, ix, 18, 45, 50, 51, 52, 53, 54, 59, 63, 65, 68, 100, 105, 111, 112, 144, 150
thorax, 4, 5, 32, 33, 40
tin, 33
tissue, 85
titanium, 92, 96, 99
tonic, 51
tooth, 65
trace elements, 141
training, 63, 85, 112
trajectory, 54
transducer, 138, 148
transduction, 155
transmission, 2, 18, 19, 20, 22, 23
transplantation, 138, 149
transport, 135
trapezius, 124
treatment methods, 102
trial, 54, 87, 156
trigeminal nerve, 56
tryptophan, 139, 154
tumor(s), 5, 145, 150, 151, 157
tumours, 96, 140, 150
Turkey, 78
turnover, 44, 93, 100
twins, 43, 142, 152

U

UK, 125, 152
United, 113
United States, 113
urine, 93
USA, 79, 105, 125

V

valve, 63
variables, ix, 55, 78, 80, 83, 84, 85, 89, 105, 115
variations, 54
velocity, 122, 123

ventilation, 71
vertebrae, 4, 6, 7, 8, 33, 34, 35, 37, 58, 141, 146, 155, 159
vertical dimensions, 55
vestibular system, 93, 121
vision, 59, 88, 89, 123

W

walking, ix, 112, 119, 122, 123, 129, 130, 133, 134, 135
weakness, 37, 38, 50, 74, 94
wear, 37, 40, 58, 60, 71
well-being, 65
wild type, 27, 28, 29
wires, 95
workers, 61
World Health Organization, 65
worldwide, viii, 91, 92, 98

X

xrays, 95
x-rays, 109, 114, 115

Y

Y chromosome, 142
young adults, 68, 71
young people, 75, 86

Z

zinc, 141, 152